WITH CHILD

Also by Phyllis Chesler

WOMEN AND MADNESS
WOMEN, MONEY AND POWER
ABOUT MEN

WITH CHILD

A Diary
of Motherhood

Phyllis Chesler

THOMAS Y. CROWELL, PUBLISHERS
Established 1834
New York

FIRST EDITION

DESIGNER: LESLIE PHILLIPS

Library of Congress Cataloging in Publication Data

Chesler, Phyllis.
  With child, a diary of motherhood.

  1. Pregnancy—Psychological aspects. 2. Childbirth—Psychological aspects. 3. Mother and child. 4. Chesler, Phyllis. 5. Mothers—United States—Biography. 6. Feminists—United States—Biography. I. Title.
RG560.C47 1979   301.41'2'0924 [B]   79–7081
ISBN 0–690–01835–5

---

79 80 81 82 83 10 9 8 7 6 5 4 3 2 1

For my son

   Ariel,

this hand-made gift,

to welcome you

Acknowledgments

My gratitude and love to Nachmy Bronstein and Laurie Juengert, who made this book possible in the most concrete and daily of ways.

My love to those friends who encouraged me during this double rite of passage, my having a baby and having a book about having a baby: Esther Broner, Z. Budapest, Jonathan Fast, Georgina Gorra, Grace Griffin, Cyrill Halkin, Marion Howard, Erica Jong, Bea Kreloff, Elaine Kaplan, Karen Lippert, Janet MacLeod, Robin Morgan, Letty Pogrebin, Connie Proto, Janet Roslund, Anne Kent Rush, Gail Spira, Gloria Steinem, Sheila Sussman, Victor Turkel.

My deep thanks to Elaine Markson, my agent, and to Arnold Dolin, my editor, for being there for me.

My thanks to Laurie Juengert, Ida Messana, Andrea Rosen and Emily Schaefer for their intelligent assistance.

My thanks to all the mothers who spent time with me— most of all, my own mother.

This is a true story, but all the names have been changed except my own, my son Ariel's and the late Margaret Mead's.

Part One

PREGNANCY

May 1, 1977

Child: How imperiously you make yourself known. This morning I vomited.

. My teeth are chattering. My fear—such fear!—seems to rise up out of history, to swirl through my bowels, all the way up to my teeth. *I'm afraid of you.* Who are you, that I tremble so?

Why am I having a baby? How many women have asked themselves this question? Am I any different, any freer, than those mothers who never asked?

I am without the hystory of female askings. I ask as if for the first time.

I've heard mothers try to talk about pregnancy, or children, in the midst of "adult" conversation. Always, they risk indifference—from others with something "larger" to say. As if an individual tale of pregnancy isn't important. As if all mothers—or children—are alike.

Little one: This journal will be a record of my askings; a record of our beginnings; a record of our awakening; a record of the fact that before you, there was me. Who in the middle of my life—in chaos—choose you.

Know that I'm terrified of the enormous responsibility.

What if I have to choose between my work and you—and can't?

What if I can't earn enough money?

What if I can't transform myself into a mother-person?

Do all women die in childbirth to be reborn as mothers? Does your coming mean my death?

Why am I having you? Do I think you'll always be there for me? Do I believe that only you, an unborn child, are my true beloved, my marriage mate, till death do us part? *I do.*

Why am I having you? Am I afraid I'd regret *not* becoming a mother? Have they finally gotten to me: those who say that all else for women is ephemeral, unsatisfying?

Have I lingered in your father's arms, these many years, just waiting for you? Can I leave him, now that you're here?

Am I bored with my work? Or is it the growing knowledge that I won't be allowed to *do* my work, that has me turning to thoughts of you?

Listen, child: I hear them at my heels. My breath grows short. I choose you to throw them off my trail. I choose you so that when I'm next accused of daring too much, of wanting too much, of having too much (for a woman), they'll pause, and see us—only a mother and child—and call off their inexorable laws.

Are *you* my cover? Can women hide behind children without becoming very small ourselves?

To embrace what has been is foreign to me. *Women have always had children. Children have always had women.* Despite this, despite everything I know, still I choose your existence. In doing this, I accept my own.

I am every woman who has dared to hope that *despite everything,* a child will sweeten her days, soften the blow of loneliness and old age.

I am every woman who has ever honored her mother by becoming a mother.

You are my emissary to the next century. You, child, are my life offering to all the mothers who have preceded me.

The great and greatly silenced Mothers. There's a shelf in my local bookstore marked "Child Care," with books by male experts on annual expected growth rates and separation anxiety; books praising natural childbirth; books damning obstetrical procedures in America. Here's a book on how to form your own child care center.

Twenty books in all.

I find a handful of precious, brave books, all published in the last five years, by mothers on motherhood. Where are the thousand descriptions of pregnancy and labor, the dreams and consequences of mother-longings in every century, every culture?

Child: I'll search for Mothers, dead and alive, to guide me. In dusty manuscripts, in new anthologies—in my living room or theirs.

*M*ay 8, 1977

On Mother's Day, at dinner, I tell my mother I'm pregnant with you. "Oh," she says, chewing slowly. "It's about time."

If my father were alive, he'd be shouting with excitement. He'd be crying. But there she sits, immovable as ever. I'm unprepared for such indifference.

I leave the restaurant, cheeks burning. How can she, of all women, not rejoice? Who, then, will rejoice with me if not my mother? Suddenly I'm returned to my childhood, to my search for mothering.

In becoming pregnant, am I hoping to find a mother rather than become one? Does a mother need a mother even more than a daughter does? But who's the mother now, who's the child?

My mother is my child. She's herself, only in child form. (Like the nineteenth-century dolls with grown-up faces.) Her peevish dependence annoys me. I'm shocked by my own coldness. I dress her. I scold her for wetting her pants. She is me when I was a child. I am her.

Oh, child, I'll have an abortion. I never want to feel such coldness toward another person. Definitely not toward you. It's better we end it now. No, I'll keep you—to spite her! In spite of her! Why should I let her come between us?

You'll be my mother, my family! (Is this why women have children?)

Baby: Your grandmother hardly ever laughed. She trusted no one, expected nothing. She was always "doing something": the dishes, the cooking, the shopping. She was either dressing one child or taking another to school.

She was always avoiding being alone with me.

Once it must have been different between us. Before my first brother was born: when there were only the two of us alone together all day, every day, for three and a half years. I can't remember having her. I only remember losing her.

*M*ay 10, 1977

Since 1971 I've received eight thousand letters from people, sharing their lives with me, asking me for advice. Whom should I write now? Who will answer my questions? Who will believe that I don't have the answers? Who will believe that I'm so scared?

Suddenly, women in the "ordinary"—mothers—seem wise to me. Mothers *must* know what I need to know. I'm going to begin asking the mothers I know all the important questions.

Will you and I love each other?

Will we *really* love each other?

What happens if we don't?

Who will mother me, so that I can mother you?

May 11, 1977

Coffee with Doris, the mother of two daughters in their teens.

"How did you do it?" I ask. "Who helped you?"

"Only my mother—and my husband when he could," she tells me. "My mother lived in my building. I could leave the baby with her when I wanted a coffee break."

"No one else helped you?"

"Phyllis, who do you expect to help you? No one helps mothers. That's what a mother does: help others."

"Oh."

She toasts me with cappuccino.

"I wonder how different things will be for you. Probably not much. But who can tell?"

May 15, 1977

Sitting on my couch, another mother. Angie married the "right" man, became rapidly pregnant in her early twenties, has three children under ten. *She* must know what I need to know.

"Who helped you?" I ask. "How did you manage so many kids all at once?"

"So you're really doing it." She smiles at me with admiration. And affection. "Who helped? *I* helped! That's it. That's the whole story. My mother made me crazy: I wouldn't let her into the hospital after I gave birth. My mother's attitude was: *I* did it alone; no reason you can't. She didn't think I should ever have a baby-sitter. *Mothers* belong at home, not strangers. My husband was busy; he helped weekends. But I was really alone for five years managing three kids."

"Swallowed up alive is that it? Never alone, but always alone?"

"Something like that," she replies cheerfully. "And, Phyllis, labor hurts like hell. Don't let them lie to you about taking deep breaths and—presto!—here's a cute baby."

"Oh."

May 17, 1977

"Darling, it's the task of Sisyphus—but what isn't? My son is a pleasure, a joy, a real companion." This is Stella speaking, a new mother twenty-five years ago.

"Once you're a mother you're always a mother, no matter how old you are or how old *they* are.

"My oldest daughter doesn't speak to me at all." She tells me this for the first time. "She hasn't for four years. Her analyst thinks I'm the original monster mother. It took me four years to stop trying to reach her. Maybe she'll never speak to me again."

"Does she see her father?" I ask.

"Not really. But she does go to him for money. She couldn't get as much from me. I can't earn as much."

Oh. Some children never speak to their mothers again. *Years have gone by when I haven't spoken to mine. . . .*

"Stella, who helped you with your children when they were very young?"

"My mother would have. She would have done everything for me. But she died three months after I got married. I had to struggle alone."

May 18, 1977

Another mother and I sit in a restaurant. Nora's son is eight years old. We touch each other in excitement.

"Phyllis, I'm so pleased! I've been wondering for a while now: which of the "early warriors" would decide to become a mother—after feminism. And it's you."

"Who helped you, Nora?"

"Help? Oh, my dear. Don't be absurd. My mother is completely impossible. And movements can't be relied on. I couldn't count on comrades with no time, who were actively hostile to children. My husband and some of his male friends were my child care support network. . . . Will you breast-feed?" she asks.

"Of course," I reply. "Sure. But how do you travel to lectures and breast-feed too?"

"Good question. You take a nasty little breast pump with you and squeeze your milk out in the lonely motel room so that your breasts don't ache—and your milk supply doesn't dry up. You try not to miss the baby too much. You try not to think that your presence is more essential than his father's. You try not to be guilty. You *avoid* losing your mind."

"Nora, I'm scared. I never thought I'd have a child."

"Relax, my love. It gets worse as you go on. *May as well get used to not being in control.*"

"Nora, tell me: why don't you have another child?"

She pauses, as if searching for an answer, as if suppressing the one at her lips.

"Phyllis, it's too hard. It's even hard to describe *how* it's too hard—and we know words don't fail me."

"Oh."

May 19, 1977

My mother just called. She doesn't mention my being pregnant. I find myself screaming. I hang up on her.

I hold my breath when the phone rings again, afraid that it's her, with something to say that will hurt me. That will hurt her. That will have us screaming at each other, hanging up in midsentence.

Why doesn't she warm toward me now that I'm pregnant?

I go to visit a Mother.

"Miriam, did you ever fight with your mother when you were pregnant?"

"Never. That was the best time. That was the only time I could do no wrong." My friend Miriam was first pregnant in 1951. "Your mother comes to visit. She looks your belly over. She brings something for you to eat, something for you to wear. She touches your hair. She smiles. Then, who do you go see on the way to the hospital? Your mother. She says: My daughter, I wish I could bear your pain for you.

"But when you're *not* pregnant, she nags, she attacks, she turns her face from you. She praises only her sons. My mother helped me with the children—but she never recognized or liked anything else I produced. My daughter the mother—never my daughter the playwright. If you want to be pampered by *my* mother, stay pregnant."

Ah, a traditional mother in 1951, in 1851, in 1751 B.C. . . . I wish she were mine. I wish my mother would crow over my belly. Did she crow over her own when I was in it? In 1940, did my grandmother pamper her before I was born? Or did sickness, poverty and so many other grandchildren prevent the crowing over my mother?

Would I behave in such a traditional way toward a pregnant daughter?

I ask every mother I can find how her mother treated

her when she was pregnant. So far, very few women have described being overprotected by their mothers when they were pregnant.

No woman seems to experience her father's absence or busyness when she's pregnant as a form of abandonment. In fact, whatever fathers do to "help out" is overly appreciated because so unexpected.

Secretly I'm sure that if my father were alive, he'd visit me at least three times a week, bearing flowers, candy. He'd take me to the zoo, to Coney Island. I believe he'd *court* me, he'd *baby* me during this pregnancy.

Why won't my mother "baby" me? Pregnant, do I remind her of the mother she never had? Does she want me to "baby" her?

Even pregnant, I don't bring out the adoring courtier in my mother. Or do I, and is my long-silent courtier spurned again, this time for a grandchild? I cast my mother aside for my father, my girlfriends, my boyfriends, and always she warned me: "I told you so," when things fell apart.

She never said: "Love me, don't leave me." She only said: "Fix your hair, act like a lady, settle down." Somewhere else.

I visit the Mothers.

Lila tells me that her mother didn't visit her until her daughter was a month old, and then just stayed for dinner.

Gudrun tells me to expect my mother to "prefer" her grandchild to me. "She'll do things for her grandchild that you never saw her do before. You won't mind this. She's the only one you'll really be able to count on for emergency baby-sitting."

Roberta describes how *her* mother suddenly became "helpless" with her grandchild, and wasn't always available to baby-sit.

Is my mother really giving notice that she's resigning her commission as my mother? Is she saying: "I don't ever want to sacrifice myself again to a child. I did that for you and now there's nothing left of me *to* give. . . ."

My mother asks, this giant of my childhood: "How do you like your tea? Should I fix my roof or not?" *She makes no promises about what I can count on when you arrive.*

Would I cheerfully leave my life to take care of a totally dependent grandmother? Wouldn't I make my resentment felt?

How little my mother thinks she's loved! How afraid she is of being scorned for doing something "wrong." How much she fears she's merely needed. How she resents it!

May 20, 1977

Who will be family to you, child of mine? What holy days will we celebrate? What memories will you have of candles lit, or of tables covered with snowy linen, around which many, many people sit? Whom will you play with and where? Will you meet people now who will know you all your life? Or like me, will you have to begin again each time?

How I long for ceremonies! For celebrations! Will this obsess me so much that eventually I'll spin another child and yet another child out of my own blood? Is this one of the reasons that women have more children?

May 21, 1977

Child: Will you have your father's beauty: his thick lashes, his dark hair? Will you have his eyes: the eyes of Rachael, the eyes of David?

Your father was born in Israel in 1950, when I was ten years old. Through him, you're a child of one of the first "legal" Jews in two thousand years. I conceived you as soon as you were historically possible. I swear, it's the last thing I'll arrange for you. As they say, "After this, I wash my hands of it."

Tell me: Are you the Messiah? How splendid, then, if you're a girl. Forget what I've just said. Your real father is a Goddess. You'll enter Jerusalem through a fifth gate—and there'll be no denying you.

I met your father, David, in the south of Israel in 1973. There, in Eilat, where the mountains are pink, the sand white; there, where you can see Jordan winking across the turquoise waters, the possibility of your existence began.

When did your life begin? Was it really in 1973, in Israel? Or was it one moment, long ago, in my childhood? In my mother's childhood—in *her* mother's childhood?

Was it written on the sky that your father was meant to please me, so that you could exist? Was he placed in my path, so casually, so perfectly, in order to tempt me, in order to gentle me into having you?

Did your existence begin when sperm met egg? Or twenty hours later, when I was alone, on an airplane, or giving a lecture?

What day, what night was it? And in what city of the world? I'm not sure. I ask your father. He's not sure either.

Did your existence begin when the urine test confirmed it? Or was it before that, when I sensed your presence in me?

Will you exist only if I go through with my pregnancy? Do you *really* exist?

May 22, 1977

Today, at a women's health-care benefit, two obstetricians fight over whether I should or shouldn't have an amniocentesis test.

"Look," says Denise. "We don't know what damage that test causes in the long run. Or what trauma it presents to the fetus."

"But Phyllis can't risk having a Mongoloid baby," Sandy insists.

"Sisters," I say, "I appreciate your concern, but please: don't speak about me as if I'm not in the room. . . ."

"Phyllis, I'm having a nervous breakdown." A newly famous writer with wild, rolling eyes clutches at me, swooning, screaming about lost friends, about hostile television hosts.

"Calm down," I tell her. "Don't take it too seriously. If you become addicted to being at the center of whirlwind attention, you'll feel dead, unloved, when it stops. Which it always does."

She clings to me but doesn't hear what I'm saying. I hug her. I bring her a drink.

"Please don't have a nervous breakdown. By the way, I'm pregnant."

It doesn't seem to register. She can only hear the sound of her own voice. I back away very quietly, wave goodbye to the still arguing physicians, and go home.

May 23, 1977

I guess I feel I should be congratulated as well as *heard* when I say I'm pregnant. Given my mother's apparent coldness, given my own terror, anything less than gladness on my behalf makes me fear for myself.

What kind of woman would withhold her verbal support for so significant a choice of mine? Why am I so sensitive about what other women think of me? Is it because pregnancy is *supposed* to signify a great bond among women, a female affirmation of womanhood, that I grow frightened, disappointed, when any woman refuses to honor this claim, for any reason? (I, who only a few months ago hardly ever noticed pregnant women or small children; I, who have spent so few evenings, or weekends, or summers, in the "company of" mothers and small children.)

Am I pregnant with you in order to be blessed by women? Am I that starved for female approval, that punished by female disapproval, that I'd endanger both of us—for the love of women?

Am I Candide, about to be duped by my own illusions: namely, that women automatically help and love pregnant women and new mothers? *Women are busy people:* especially if they're mothers. Especially if they're not mothers.

Where, then, is our tribe of powerful female elders sitting beside the sea—pounding spices, exchanging stories, singing? Not in New York City. Not in the twentieth century. Whereabouts unknown to my circle.

Can I ask Carolyn to put off lobbying for the Equal Rights Amendment, in order to sit with me, feel your kicks, allay my anxieties?

Can I ask Nora to put off writing poems, put off earning a living, put off taking care of her own child, in order to be a daily sister in my house?

Can I ask Constance to stop seeing patients, stop lecturing, turn down academic panels and all emergencies, so that she'll be available if I happen to need her?

Can I ask Miriam to leave her husband and three children, bring her plays and all her jewelry, move in with me and be my mother?

Can I even ask myself to stop my life because you're joining it?

May 24, 1977

Last month, filled with intimations of immortality, I eased myself up onto my friend Constance's examining table and asked her to confirm your existence. She palpated, began to smile:

"Phyllis, if you're going to have a baby, it might as well be now. You're definitely pregnant."

"Joker!" I managed to laugh. "Will you kick in some money for diapers and higher education?"

"Sure," she said. "What's one more loan to me?"

What banterers we are. We gossip and laugh so much together that I never feel she's a "doctor": an expert whose knowledge and experience are beyond my reach. There is no way to describe what it feels like to have women friends who are doctors, lawyers, accountants, architects, carpenters, poets, teachers, politicians, nurses. . . . To be able to call an "expert" who is also a friend, and not the business acquaintance of a husband or father, is as close as I come to feeling safe, powerful.

Constance's hands are large and very soft. I'd love her to deliver you, but she doesn't deliver babies anymore. I fantasize that she'll arrive with a black doctor's bag. We'll have dinner together. At the necessary moment we'll lay our conversation aside—and have a baby!

Maybe I should share my fantasy with her. Maybe it's her fantasy too. *What if it's not?* So I say nothing and decide to visit Frédéric, my "official" gynecologist of ten years.

May 27, 1977

In the last ten years, Frédéric has climbed down mountains, met me in emergency rooms on early Sunday mornings, performed an abortion for me in 1972, with sad, silent eyes. I choose Frédéric—because he cares about me, respects me. He knew me long before I became "known" for my views. He is like a family friend, a relative. I trust him. He is one of the gentle men.

Frédéric's expensive. *You're* expensive. It will cost one thousand dollars to have you with his help. This includes all prenatal obstetrical checkups and delivery itself. This *doesn't* include the cost of prenatal tests: an amniocentesis test, urine and blood tests, ultrasound tests; and any prescribed medication. One thousand dollars doesn't include the cost of the hospital room, the delivery room, hospital medication, the cost of nurses if they're needed. A Caesarean costs five hundred dollars: extra.

My medical plan covers the cost of the hospital room, but only two hundred fifty dollars of Frédéric's fee, and a small portion of all the tests. All together, it will cost about five thousand dollars to have you as a middle-class baby in 1977.

Nuclear weapons are public responsibilities. Babies are each woman's frivolity, each family's private responsibility.

I want a midwife. I offer Frédéric the option of being my midwife.

"How many labors and deliveries have you ever assisted from start to finish, Frédéric? Do you have a sweet singing voice? Will you massage my feet and be there for me? If so, I choose you as my midwife!"

Frédéric looks thoughtful, almost wistful.

"What if I have emergency surgery, and you're in an early stage of labor?" he parries.

"What if, indeed," I say. "So we'll find me a midwife."

If I have a midwife, will they fight over who delivers the baby? Is that an "issue"? Is actual delivery a prize?

*M*ay 31, 1977

Pamela at dinner: Loving and funny, she tells me the details of "leaving" her two sons sixteen years ago, when they were three and four years old.

"I left my husband and took them both with me. I had to leave our house because he wouldn't. I moved into a cheap room in the neighborhood. I hadn't finished college when I got married, so my ways of earning money were limited. My parents wouldn't help, partly because they couldn't, partly because they *wouldn't*. They thought I was crazy, leaving a husband who earned money. I went on welfare and started job hunting. I hadn't felt so good since I got married."

"Pamela, I always thought you *wanted* to leave your kids."

She grows very quiet and slowly, very slowly, says:

"Oh, no. My husband refused to give me any money. My parents were on his side. He offered to take the boys totally, or insisted that I move back. I went crazy—literally—for a year and a half. I got jobs, I left jobs, I had two kids under five. You don't know what that means yet.

"I only wanted help with them. I didn't want to leave them: definitely not in the hands of their father. *But I was totally alone.* It became me or them. When I knew I'd kill myself, I decided to try life. I let him have the boys—only until I could get on my feet. I visited every weekend."

"What happened?" It's deathly still between us now.

"He agreed to a divorce—if he had total custody. He had a new wife lined up. His lawyer was ugly with me. He'd present me as such a bad mother, as so crazy, as such a lunatic lesbian communist free-lover, that no judge would even give me visitation rights. I caved in. *It was 1965. . . .*

"I visited. I visited them. But each week they were turned against me more. It moved from 'Mommy, why did you leave us' to 'Mommy, you're not a good person for us' to 'We don't want to talk to you.'

"We haven't talked to each other for ten years. I wrote to them. The letters always came back unopened. Last year I tried to see my oldest son. He refused. And his father had a lawyer send me a threatening letter if I ever approached him again. . . ."

So: you can be taken away by fathers and their new wives; you can be taken away if I'm poor, or if I refuse to be a "wife." You can be taught to hate me if I'm forced to abandon you.

This is too chilling. Maybe I should leave your father now, flee to some place where this can never happen. Now, now do I understand the silence of mothers, the conservatism of mothers: the craftiness of women.

To think that child custody for mothers is as recent and as fragile a right as higher education is for women! To think that a father legally owns his children—and can use this as a threat over a mother, as a form of blackmail—and can win custody if he's determined to do so. And can marry a new wife to perform the daily child care. And be praised for caring so much about his own children; praised for rescuing them from their own mother.

Tonight—can you sense it?—we sleep far over on our side of the bed.

June 3, 1977

Child: *Your father is not afraid of me. Therefore, you exist.* Not once in four years did he abandon me to my strength, or demand that I choose between my work and him. More: he knows how to leave me alone. (I need to be left alone— *but by somebody.*)

Child: your father is mother, father, brother, sister to me. He is my family body: warm, familiar, in my bed. In sickness and in health, always and long after friends have left for the night, or for good, he is here.

Rare. Priceless—not without cost. We argue in closed, moving cars, a-seethe with boredom. I wonder, he wonders, if our "different" relationship isn't too hard, isn't killing us both—slowly, inevitably. We make wild accusations.

I miss him terribly when I'm on the road, call home once or twice a day just to hear his voice: "How are you? Did you take your vitamins? How's school, are you constipated? Where were you last night? Do you miss me, I miss you . . ."

Child: What if *you* come between us?

June 4, 1977

Helen is the mother of a twenty-four-year-old son. I "interview" her on motherhood.

"I think it's splendid you're having a baby," she says. "I stayed with my husband all those years just for my son's sake. Well, for my sake too. I was too scared to be alone. I thought a boy needed his father. I still do. Although fathers can be awfully rough on sons. . . .

"Listen, Phyllis, a child is worth it. Husbands come and go. They're not really there for you, if you know what I mean. But a child! If you're there now for a child, that child is always there for you."

I've heard mothers say this before. Is it true? After all, *I'm* not "always there" for my mother.

June 6, 1977

Dinner with Silvana. She's telling me how lonely she is, how much she'd love some loving.

"What happened to the men, Phyllis? Is it like this for everyone else? Good sex with married men only—*if* you're not married to them? And the arguments about whether to live together or not, whether to "make a commitment" or not! And watch out if they "give in." They expect royal treatment: gratefulness, breakfast in bed. I don't know. Maybe it's New York. Maybe it's American men over forty. Maybe it's me."

"Silvana," I say tentatively, afraid of what I'm going to suggest. "Silvana, have you ever thought that the kind of love relationship you fantasize about isn't possible with a grown man, but only with a child? Or only with an entire social community? Or only with a great ideal? Maybe what women need is enough money to support a child, a really decent job, lots of female friends, good lovers—and a child for romance, for a lifetime commitment."

"But I want a man who'll give me all that. That's why I want a man."

"Maybe they can't give us 'all that.' Maybe they have nothing to do with 'all that.' Maybe your men over forty are angry, withholding, because you're asking them for what they haven't got. And they're guilty about it."

"But how can I have a baby without someone to help me?"

"Some*one*? As far as I can figure, every mother needs at least four mothers *for herself*, so she can mother one baby. And men aren't too good in the mothering department."

I wonder, baby, how "romantic" I'll be about you when I'm tired, when I'm depressed, when I've had it with 3 A.M. feedings, doctor bills, screams to quiet, and the responsibility for it all, which won't go away.

My mother did it for me. I'll make sure, somehow, that you're always dry and clean and fed and warm, and . . .

How? How will I make sure? Will I do it myself—and give up my own life for a while? Will I be able to pay someone to do it for me? What if this "someone" is a child-molester? A heavy, hostile presence in our life?

What if your father won't really take care of you?

"Silvana, don't get pregnant too quickly," I say. "It's a complex proposition—this 'love' we say we must have, this 'love' we say we'll die without."

June 12, 1977

Charlotte is forty-two this month. She's going to Italy for the summer. When I tell her I'm pregnant, she looks away.

"Oh, congratulations, by all means congratulations," she says, sharply, falsely.

"Charlotte, what is it?"

"Phyllis, I've been trying to get pregnant for three years. I'm not going to use any birth control in Italy."

"But how can you afford, emotionally, to have a baby alone? Your apartment is just big enough for *you*," I joke.

"Oh." She laughs shortly, toughly. "I'll find a place for a baby. It's no big deal."

Charlotte has lived alone since I've known her: eight years now. Every relationship she's had with a man is sexually dramatic, emotionally tumultuous—and never leads to their living together.

Is every woman over thirty-five without a child asking herself whether or not to have a child now? Is every mother of teen-agers asking herself what to do about her life now that the children are grown?

June 13, 1977

"Phyllis, you'll regret this." Meg, my friend of ten years, is yelling at me, smoking fiercely, drinking hard. "Don't do this to yourself! You have more troubles than you can handle right now. A woman writer shouldn't have a child. You'll stop writing."

Embarrassed, furious, I try to tease her out of such bad humor. I, who should have my hand held for me, my hair stroked for me by her, have to calm *her* down. Doesn't she think I'm worried about this myself?

"Simmer down, Meg, it's my problem. Why such bad temper? Do you think I plan to imprison you as the baby-sitter?"

Is it the alcohol? Does she feel I'm rejecting her some-how? Can she *possibly* be jealous? Or is she telling me that "they" won't let me get away with this; that I'll pay too high a price? Does she view the pregnancy of a woman warrior, a woman artist, as capitulation, as defeat?

What if she's right?

Baby: You may "ruin" my creative life, but like every-thing that has been important to me, you'll change it. Once, I lived each year of ten, waiting for an enormous social birth. And it happened! The bloody, painful howls of it still fill my days, every day. If that birth—the consciousness of women—hadn't happened, you probably wouldn't exist.

I wouldn't have had the courage to become a mother.

June 14, 1977

Lisa just called to tell me that she's six months pregnant. I haven't seen her since 1971, when our feminist consciousness-raising group broke up. I congratulate her, over and over. I'm afraid to tell her I'm pregnant too. I don't want her to have to share the limelight with me. We arrange to meet for coffee later today. . . .

She's glisteningly pregnant. I ask to see her naked belly. A pregnant woman is high-bellied, large-breasted: utterly beautiful.

"Lisa, how's your painting going?"

"Honestly, Phyllis, I can't concentrate on it. I'm so excited about the baby. I'm knitting and baking a lot of bread, and buying wonderful little things. . . . I walk a lot. I guess waiting is all I can do."

"Lisa, I'm pregnant too," I confide.

"But why? You don't have to . . ." she blurts out. She recovers her innate sense of decency. She smiles at me. "But of course you'd want a baby. You've been married so much longer than I have."

June 15, 1977

I'm on a panel about Women and Judaism. I sit next to Beatrice, next to Sharon, in a well-carpeted apartment filled with European survivors, American Zionists, writers, socialists, rabbis, psychiatrists, feminists, wives and husbands.

Something I've said—I can't imagine what—has gotten a man with a loud voice very upset. He's yelling at me. He can't stop himself from creating a "scene."

"Young lady," he screams at me in a British accent, "why don't you go back where you belong? I've never heard such blasphemous raving in all my life! Women rabbis indeed! Women gods! What you need is a good strong beating. Who invited you to speak anyway?"

"Frank, she's pregnant," a woman whispers. "Get hold of yourself."

"Pregnant? Why? Hasn't she done enough damage already?"

Another opinion enters the hush. "Phyllis, as a feminist, why even bother with religion? It's religion that allows Jewish capital to enslave Jewish labor in a free Jewish state." A socialist Zionist begins to make a speech.

"Phyllis, as a feminist, why be concerned with Israel at all? It's as much a patriarchal nation-state as anywhere else."

"Phyllis, the only issue is anti-Semitism. All the rest of this claptrap is a way of avoiding the problem."

A young Orthodox rabbi and his wife invite me to spend a Sabbath with them. A young man wearing a headband and shorts tells me that what I've said about ritual has "moved him" deeply.

"Phyllis," says a psychiatrist, "people can't hear what you say. It's too threatening. These things can only be dealt with on the couch. Why don't you go into practice?"

Child: Welcome to the Jewish community.

June 16, 1977

Philadelphia, a Conference on Battered Women: I listen to a young mother, wearing dark glasses, describe her husband's pattern of abuse.

"Whenever I'd get pregnant he'd go for my stomach, kick me there, forget about my face. . . ."

I can't believe what I'm hearing. Of course it's true. I've read the reports, the statistics, the interviews. I'm here to give a speech on the "phenomenon." I listen hunched over, hiding my belly with my whole upper body. I think: Not all men, only a few men; the psychopaths, the exceptions.

A second woman describes how her two sons beat her up regularly, for money. A third says it was her adolescent daughter who terrified her and then began to hit her. A fourth woman describes how the police always believed her husband. A fifth woman weeps because her family blamed her for not being able to control her husband's violence. A sixth woman explains that her husband's family warned her that if she left him he'd kill himself for sure, her kids would be orphans, and that they'd all turn their backs on the "whole mess." On and on, the women bear witness to their extraordinary powerlessness: their loyalty to their children *no matter what.*

Child: Can you hear this? Do you wonder why I've summoned you here? Do you think we can escape human evil? Do you think I can protect you from it? By closing my eyes and staying home with you, as these mothers tried to do?

June 20, 1977

The word "pregnancy," as I repeat it aloud, still bears the weight of female fear and punishment.

"Pregnancy"—as in: Did she do it? Is it "legal"? "Pregnant"—as in: misshapen, swollen. Maybe it's Rosemary's baby in there. "Pregnant"—as in a physical disease, requiring hospitalization.

Today I went to a maternity store.

Maternity clothes. Those dreadfully "cute" or resignedly serviceable garments. Should I insist upon non-sexist maternity clothes? They have them! Denim coveralls, studded jeans, lumberjack shirts, mixed in with the little-girl pinafores, the sturdy shirtwaist dresses. Who can afford to buy a full season's worth of maternity clothes? You do eventually give birth, don't you, and then you can't wear these clothes anymore. . . .

What I'd like to wear, my baby, is a hundred-breasted, thousand-jeweled garment of sapphire; a great coat of many colors; disposable gowns flecked with fake precious metals. Large, exotic clothes, to loudly and gorgeously proclaim your passage into being.

Where can I buy such clothes? Where can I wear such clothes?

June 23, 1977

I envy men their wives, those loyal, efficient women: women who sing to green plants, whose salad dressing is always perfect, who pack suitcases for other people.

I'll place an ad in the newspaper for a wife. Sex not required, salary plus benefits. I'll give her all my money. I'll always say thank you. I'll come home to good smells, Mozart playing, a table already set. The clothes from the cleaners will be hanging in my closet.

I need a slave. Who doesn't?

I've asked David many times to please bring home a wife for us. We cling to each other, siblings in a storm. What will happen with your visitation? Will *you* be our wife? Or will we be three siblings in search of a mother?

July 10, 1977

It's hard to say, "By the way, I'm pregnant." Nothing prepares me for some of the responses I get. One woman, a "friendly" acquaintance, grinned grimly at me.

"Wait and see. You won't be so high and mighty anymore. *I* was depressed for a solid year after I gave birth. This will bring you down to earth."

How will it profit her if I'm "brought down"? Will it help her to love herself more?

In Albany today, some anti-ERA and anti-abortion women yelled at me: "Don't you think it's unfair to a child to have such an old mother, and a feminist radical too!" Middle-aged ladies in nylon stockings and neat Sunday clothes they were. How easily they could shave my head for sleeping with enemy soldiers; how easily stone me for adultery; how smugly they could burn me for a witch.

"So you're really not that much of a feminist after all," said one woman on the way back from Albany. "You're just like me—a coward!" (A coward? This is one of the bravest things I've ever done.)

An old friend, grown distant because of my notoriety, called tonight to tell me she hated me. "You're going to have everything. Do you know that I've been trying to get pregnant for two years and can't? What did you do: snap your fingers?"

A pregnant woman is one's own mother pregnant with oneself. A pregnant woman is a visibly sexual creature who excites deep emotions in other women: fear, envy, pity—and a great urge to touch the swelling.

Oh, child, where is our brass band? Where is our parade? Where is *my* faery godmother? Where is the older woman to initiate me? Where are the ceremonies to welcome me into the circle of mothers? Has New York City banned such welcomings? Should I move to some other place? Some other century?

July 12, 1977

Last night I dreamed I gave birth to a monster. Are you that menacing creature I saw in my dream? My monster, myself.

I dream of our animal past. Great lizards, growly lions. World swimmers, jungle experts. Why feel horror at being joined to such a magnificent chain of life?

I guess I'll go through with the amniocentesis test.

Frédéric examined me today. I listened to your heartbeat for five full minutes. What an incredible thump and whoosh it is, little ancestor.

July 20, 1977

Mara is talking about her abortion again. The abortion
she didn't want, but had because her husband refused to
take joint responsibility for a child.

"If you want to handle it alone, then go ahead, I won't
stop you, he says. He won't stop me! *He* already has a child.
I have none. None. Now I'll never have any. Never. Never.
I'll always be an orphan."

"Why don't you have a baby anyway, if it means that
much to you?"

"I can't do it on my own. I'm too nervous, I'm too hysterical. We don't have enough money. He pays child support
as it is. Rothschild we're not."

Child, I've had four abortions. I could have been the
mother of an eighteen-year-old, a sixteen-year-old, a four-
teen-year-old, a seven-year-old. And who would I be? Would
I be myself? *Would it matter if I weren't?*

Yes, it would. How much harder it would have been
for me with a child to wrench myself out of poverty, self-
hatred. Could I have been mother to myself if I'd had children?

How lucky for both of us that I was able to act with
such resolve each time—although the fear was great, the ugli-
ness of "illegal" abortions shameful beyond recall.

July 22, 1977

Today is the amniocentesis test, a procedure routinely performed on all "elderly" gynecological patients—women over thirty-five. After looking over the release I must sign, I nearly bolt the hospital. The form says that the test results may be incorrect or accidentally "spoiled" in the laboratory; that the procedure itself is highly experimental and may induce a spontaneous miscarriage; and that knowing this, I agree never to sue and to pay their fee no matter what happens.

I'm scared. But the incidence of Mongolism is higher among women in my "age range" than is the incidence of miscarriage accidentally induced by this laboratory procedure.

How would I feel if that huge syringe—I see it lying there on the operating table—were an instrument of death? I want to leave. But what if you're Mongoloid? I lie on the table, look at the ceiling, hide my fear with scientific questions. "Oh, so the Navy developed this use of sound waves through water. How interesting!" (The water here is in my about-to-burst bladder. I've painfully and slowly hauled myself up on the table, knowing that I'll pee unendingly, any minute now.)

There you are: my baby, in me. The sonogram screen is filled with this tiny, oh, so tiny creature, floating, turning, always moving, inside my womb, alive on the three-dimensional gridded screen, alive for seventeen weeks now. I am seized with sadness! Here you are, yet to be born, yet to live, and you're being watched by so many strangers. It seems like a gross invasion of privacy. You could be a fetus in a bottle filled with formaldehyde, pickled, already born dead. You could be a visitor from another planet, trapped in a time warp, sighted on this screen in outer space.

I lie on the operating table, my belly exposed. When

the doctors find the right spot to enter with their long reverse-syringe needle, I see, *and they see,* that this baby, you, quickly move to that exact chosen spot—as if you're playing with us, as if you want no invasion.

It's over. They have my amniotic fluid. I insist on having a black-and-white picture of you. (I tell the doctors I need it for the family album.) Later, I ask people if they want to see a picture of you—and they think I'm crazy. I stare at your picture. It helps me summon you up live, turning, gravityless in space. I call it "Still Life of an Approaching World."

Did you ever notice, little star, that from a plane the earth looks like the inside of a computer: neatly divided up into squares by shiny ribbons of yellow, red, blue? In our century, nature imitates technology, not art. . . . And technology reveals awesome natural beauty, far beyond the capacity of the human eye: our own magnified body cells, distant galaxies, the movements of sea creatures. You appear to me in sound waves, moving through water. A child, forming.

July 23, 1977

The streets a-bloom with pregnant women. They stand next to me in elevators. I see them on movie lines, getting out of taxicabs, choosing fruit and vegetables. Are we invisible to everyone else? Were they here before I was pregnant? Will they all disappear when I give birth? After that, will I only notice new mothers and new babies?

*A*ugust 2, 1977

Child, your mother isn't sensible. She wants to travel while she's still single; before we meet, while I can still control things.

I'm in search of a Mother, child. For you, or for me: it's the same thing now. We're going to Crete, to Jerusalem, on a pilgrimage to find her. Maybe Rachael, your paternal grandmother, will turn Biblical, pile her belongings on her head, follow me back to New York. Maybe one of the painted Minoan women will silently come alive, leave the island with us.

An unprecedented heat wave in Athens! I'm bloated, puffy-eyed. I have diarrhea, swollen ankles, spreading feet. But I don't feel pregnant. (How do I know I don't?) The more I swell, the more *removed* I feel from my body. I'm wind, fire: no longer earth. You, child, are Nature: I am Soul. Split, still.

Only an *outsider* would conclude that all of me is involved in this physical transformation. A part of me has taken this pregnancy back at least a dozen times. A part of me has imagined you already here—and gone—a hundred times. Why am I still pregnant, then?

"I" don't believe you exist. "I" know it's only a dream. The pregnancy plods on, unmoved by my disbelief. Me, a mother? Me, have a baby?

This gross spreading of my feet: my will to root on earth.

August 3, 1977

I want David to see the Acropolis, before it's too late. Jet plane vibrations have shaken the foundations of the Parthenon. Scaffolding is everywhere. Hundreds upon hundreds of tourists step gingerly onto gangplanks, across wooden walkways.

I sit down and look at the city below. Everywhere, tiled rooftops shimmer in the haze.

What did the ancient Athenian women do when they were pregnant in such heat? Did the daughters of wealth get carried on the shoulders of pregnant servants, closer to the mountains, closer to the sea? What about the pregnant servants? What did they do with their children?

I limp through the Plaka at high noon, looking for a gift for you. I buy a small goatskin rug. Something for the house. Something to remember the Mothers of Athens by.

*A*ugust 4, 1977

Luck! If we hurry, there are two seats available on a flight to Crete. The only hotel "room" is a whitewashed *Zorba the Greek* cottage on the shore of the Aegean, in Áyios Nikó-laos. Cretan light: fierce white, tempered by the blues of ocean and sky, fresh with sea-wind. To think that no artist has painted here for fourteen hundred years!

I sit on some rocks and cool my feet in Homer's sea. I watch the sun set over the cafés, the swaying fishing boats.

Crete exists only for tourists. Where do Cretans go for vacations? What will happen to Crete when the industrial countries have no means of mass escape? Will these new, expensive hotels sink beneath the sea, to be discovered two thousand years from now? By whom?

All night, discotheque music blasts open across the Aegean. I stay awake with you. I light a candle. Child: Can you sense the moon, these waters?

*A*ugust 5, 1977

The early-morning heat is intense. My ankles are very swollen. I limp slowly, methodically, up and down the excavated levels of the Palace of Knossos. The frescoes are extraordinary. Look, child: The graceful bull-leapers are about your size and color—dark maroon, defying gravity.

Here, Mothers, I whisper, here is your daughter Phyllis, pregnant in her thirty-seventh year. How cool are your breezes, how fair thy dwelling. I linger, I linger among your columns, among your poplars.

Your goddesses, no longer in use, are shut up behind glass in the Heraklion Museum. They're surprisingly small and very personal, very endearing. I'd love to steal one: maybe the Daughter Goddess holding the snakes, maybe the Mother Goddess with her full-poured skirt. What a trial I'd have: "Pregnant Woman Steals Museum Relics for Fertility Rites, Sentenced to Mockery."

August 6, 1977

I'm gaining weight rapidly, thirty pounds already. I lumber, like an astronaut on the moon. My feet are one shoe size larger than before you existed. My breasts are huge. (I probably won't have any milk!) My calves have nearly doubled in width.

This afternoon, by the pool, a Dutchman tried to interest me in an afternoon of sex. I think he's crazy. "I'm nearly five months pregnant," I tell him. "Ah, that's interesting." He smiles. "Do you think I'd be able to see the baby? Will you let me look?" "Keep away from me: I'm a married woman . . ." *Have I really said this?*

Do I think I'm an untouchable Madonna? Do I think being pregnant is unattractive? Why? After all, I'm certainly not afraid of becoming pregnant . . .

August 7, 1977

We saw *Electra* tonight. What a betrayal of a mother by a daughter! I couldn't sit still. I paced the darkened field behind the open-air theater. What a defeat is being reenacted; on Crete, of all places! Of course, on Crete.

Oh child! What if you're a girl, and you cleave to men and men's laws, and not to me, your mother? I'll throw myself on the point of my sword.

What if you're a daughter and, like me, you hold yourself too cheaply?

What if you find my ambitions futile, my dreams embarrassing, my contradictions hypocritical?

What if I can't protect you, as my mother couldn't protect me?

Did my mother ever have such thoughts about me?

What if you're a boy, and you uphold men's laws against me, your mother?

What if you're a boy and you never leave me?

Do other pregnant women have such thoughts?

August 10, 1977

We've been bumped from the flight from Athens to Tel Aviv. They've put us up at a cardboard motel right next to takeoffs and landings. When I complain, the airlines official laughs at me. "You should be quiet," he says. "In your condition, we can have the doctor forbid you to travel." He smiles a gold-tooth smile. "Then you stay in Athens—you give birth here."

This night, here, in this terrible little motel, at 2 A.M., I have my first bout, ever, with heartburn. I actually think I'm dying. I grow hysterical. Your father forces me to drink some milk. It helps.

So you're really in there—growing hair, they tell me.

August 11, 1977

Your first kicks feel like cramps, in the airport at Athens. I think I'm having a miscarriage. I scan the crowd for a mother. A woman from Cyprus, holding a one-year-old child, tells me to "not worry," that it's only you, practicing butterfly kicks. "Enjoy it, *ma chérie*," she tells me.

What a far-flung sisterhood this is! Mothers—strangers—who talk to each other anywhere, in the language of such urgent familiarity. Will I now find it easier to talk with women about bellies than about freedom?

Ah, we're landing now, in the land of magical Sabbaths. Rachael, your Israeli grandmother, has brought us a bouquet of fresh wet flowers. And now we're drinking thick coffee by the sea, laughing, the dusk settling around us.

I can never walk the shore here without seeing the boats trying to land "illegally." I see people scrambling, swimming, being shot at; I hear their cries. This very beach in Tel Aviv was where your father and I first kissed, just back together from Eilat.

August 13, 1977

Your aunt is in the maternity hospital, dull with pain. She tries not to cry in front of me and my belly. She has just given birth to a two-pound, twenty-four-week-old girl by emergency Caesarean. The child lives: a tiny mechanical doll, hooked up to ten different machines and recording devices. I stare at her for a long while. Her face is not clearly shaped yet. You're a month younger than she is. You're even more of a monster.

A maternity hospital is not where I belong right now. The women are moaning. The heat is overwhelming. Suddenly I fear for your life. Are you still alive? Did I kill you with traveling? Despite a long line of waiting women, I persuade a nurse to persuade a doctor to listen to your heartbeat—right away. What if there is none? I'll tear my belly open with grief. I'll turn into a pillar of salt. I'll forget you ever existed.

"Everything is fine, just fine," the harassed doctor says. And I listen to your fast nonstop amplified heartbeat, the most comforting electronic sound I've ever heard. I'd like to just lie there and keep listening, to calm myself down, to reassure myself that life is as commonplace an occurrence as death.

I hear a woman giving birth. I talk to a restless and wild-eyed woman who stops to tell everyone she's in her *tenth month* of pregnancy, and "nothing doing." The place feels like a female psychiatric ward, a brothel; like ladies' day at the Turkish baths.

August 14, 1977

I want to have orgasms without foreplay three or four times every day. I look at your father slyly, passively. I insist he come back to bed, "now." If we're outside, I suggest we borrow a friend's bedroom, or sneak into a hotel restroom, "for just a minute."

I am without shame. Never have I been in such sexual heat. Is this natural in pregnancy? Or am I enjoying my lust because I think it unnatural, taboo? What exactly is so arousing, so pleasurably "lewd" to me about a woman with a round, fat belly initiating orgasms in Mediterranean heat? Is my body remembering something? Can bodies do this?

No one—not my mother, not my obstetrician, no book— has told me that you might demand orgasms the same way you demand food and oxygen: insistently, elementally, without asking my permission.

What if I were alone now? What if your father weren't obliging? What if I were forbidden to name or act upon what I'm feeling?

During, and after, love-making I watch my stomach, I watch you, like a voyeur, as if I'm not present. There's a direct line from my *consciousness* of your existence to my clitoris. Watching my belly, having my belly seen by another, seems to throb this mysterious line awake.

My serpent rises lazily, a full four feet, then coils back into its clitoral hood. My tiger is gone, my tiger returns, restless, ready to prowl again.

The fleshpots of the Middle East . . . a small room with a balcony. Long afternoons. Late mornings. The Tropic of Pregnancy.

August 15, 1977

Visions in orgasm. Babies, mysterious with Mona Lisa smiles. Hundreds of tiny Cupids, Cupid-clouds really, above my head. Don't drift away! My pleasure must pluck one of you down into me forever.

Lilith and her succulent minion of babes: how dutifully fecund of her! To fly so gloriously at prayer surrounded by hundreds and thousands of infants: angel gifts in search of mothers.

What richness in my blood, what heat in my clitoris, to sense, to imagine, each of my orgasms enclosing a pregnancy, enclosing a hundred pregnancies.

How female a sexual fantasy. The lust of mysticism, the lust of immortality.

A painted woman is dancing for me. Hips, belly, breast, circling my desire. Circe, you tempt me, you understand me.

August 16, 1977

Tamar is a thirty-eight-year-old "unwed" mother. She breast-feeds her daughter in a maple rocking chair, hair disheveled, eyes soft.

"The labor was terrible—wasn't it, my soul?—but the doctor was so good, wasn't he good?" She croons these words to her baby. Her exposed breast is wonderfully round, her nipple huge, dark.

"Tamar, how did you manage to set yourself up?" Admiringly I move around her small apartment, filled with plants and books, with all the necessary baby furniture, kitchen utensils.

"My sister helped. My aunt flew from Paris to be with me when I gave birth. And the women of Jerusalem! One brought a crib. Another gave me baby clothes. Someone brought toys. Everyone encouraged me, supported me. Little by little, everything will work out. I'll become the mistress of a rich old man; who knows?"

I don't think I'd have the courage, the foolishness, to do what she's doing. She's totally dependent on the charity, the whims, of strangers. How long can the gift-giving last? What will she do for money? Whom will she ultimately snare to "mother" the baby so that she can rejoin her dance troupe?

Tamar seems at peace with herself. She laughs easily, often. Maybe she's gone mad? How can she live with so many unknowns? So what if the apartment is dark, dirty? So what if she looks as if she hasn't slept in three months? (She probably hasn't.) *So what if I couldn't write in this setting?* Clearly, she's flourishing.

August 19, 1977

I've just called New York. You're a boy! It's late Friday afternoon. A holy quiet has begun in the city. I go to the Wailing Wall and press my stomach against it. Idly, perversely, I think to go to the men's side, claiming my rightful presence there. I contain a male child. They'd probably stone me to death.

Hear, O Israel, I am One. Mother and Child. Male and Female. Past and Future. My belly warms the sun-glown stones.

But you're supposed to be a girl! You're supposed to be just like me, only more so. I'm shocked that you come to me in male form, little self. Has ever a mother wavered over the fact that her first born will be a boy? *Will you hate me for thinking these thoughts? Can you already feel what I'm thinking?*

Ah, you're lucky, little baby. For you there is no hundred-year program ready. I'm terrified of what some women might feel about my having a son.

Before women I stand accused. It pleases me to have a son.

A conversation:

Me: I'm a little nervous about having a boy.

Your father: Phyllis, if you were having a girl, how would you feel?

Me: Nervous.

Your father: Well, I guess you're nervous about having a baby. Calm down. Maybe you'll have something else. . . .

But what of that other, darker matter: the having of a daughter whom you want to be the mother your mother never was to you, and her wanting you to be the mother you can never be to her, and the years it takes to work it out . . . that tragic dialogue I am temporarily spared by you.

August 20, 1977

Tonight Hava took us to an "open house" at Ada's. What a Great Mother Ada is! A pioneer from Russia in 1905; still setting up her samovar for new Russian immigrants, pouring tea, giving comfort. I never want to leave her.

"Ada," I tell her, "I would have gone back to Russia, to Poland, to Rumania. I would have died there in the snow. It's too hot for me here. Forget about crop failure, swamp malaria, Arab raids, British occupation; my ideological fervor would have been wiped out by a single summer, pregnant."

"Little one," she answers me, "you would have stayed. Believe me, it's never been so hot as it is right now. And you're pregnant, you're without your mother, you have no group, you're running around. You know, you don't look so good. Alexei!" She calls over one of the many men seated in the living room circle. "She has some fever, no?"

I do. I definitely am coming down with "something." But I stay until 3 A.M., caught up in the sweetness of these old-worldly exiles sitting together in Jerusalem.

"You should come and live here," Ada says. "You can make something happen. In America, what can you do? What can you do as a Jew?"

How did the pregnant Jewish slaves in Egypt survive slavery—and such heat?

August 21, 1977

Outside, it's 110 degrees. Pioneers, sabras, are fainting in the streets. They're being carried off to hospitals. I lie here on a mattress, without air conditioning, without a breeze, and look listlessly at the Judean mountains. I long for snow in New England, for white steeples, for cool forests, for blessedly crisp autumns, for light-hearted springs. (In America, I long for Jerusalem the Golden.)

Child: I'm plagued with infections—an ear infection from the Aegean, and now a stomach flu. Whom have I offended to be so cursed?

Mornings, for two days now, I throw up. I sleep by day, toss by night. I have diarrhea. Is this a virus or malaria? I'm too weak to get off the mattress. I'm dizzy, nauseous.

The women find me. They bring their questions, their demands, to my mattress. *They don't seem to see that I'm wretched with sickness. Their hunger is too great. Is this what being a mother is like?* How do you start a rape counseling center? What about a shelter for battered women? How do you deal with the violent husbands? Are there any shelters for prostitutes in America? What are the women doing about equal rights in America? What do they know about women in Israel? Is it always so hard to start a women's street theater group, publishing house, living collective? What books *must* be read? How can you tell if a psychologist is a woman-hater or not? A gynecologist? Your husband? What do you do if he is? On and on and on.

I would return to New York tonight if I could. I can't. I can't afford to forfeit my charter flight ticket. Will I die here? Have I contracted some exotic, lingering disease? ("Phyllis was never the same after her last trip to the Orient.")

A friend brings a doctor. He gives me pills which make me throw up violently. "Don't take any more," he instructs me by phone, and hangs up. (Well, I *am* in the Middle East.)

*A*ugust 22, 1977

Your father takes care of me as only a mother would do. He worries over me. He cools my forehead. He watches me sleep. He coaxes me into eating.

I'm jealous of the time he spends with his family. I'm ashamed of myself. I'm annoyed, frightened, when he's gone too long, visiting old friends. I weep, tell him I'm afraid of fainting, afraid of being left alone. "I'm out of my element here," I explain. Do I mean my work-routines, or my usual "element" of not being pregnant?

Is this why I'm so sick? To keep him by my side, to turn him into a mother—so that I can be a baby?

What price shall I have to pay for so much forbidden mothering? What terrible price?

August 24, 1977

Something terrible is happening. Frédéric just called me from New York.

"Phyllis, it's nothing important, but listen to me carefully. Go to Hadassah Hospital, to the Cytogenetics Department. Tell them that the baby has giant or satellite cells in the D-15 group of chromosomes. They must take blood from both you and David."

"Frédéric, what does this mean? Exactly? I'll take ten blood tests, happily—but what's the significance of satellite cells?"

"Probably nothing, but just do as I say."

Within one hour, straight from my sick-mattress, we're having tea with the assistant chief of cytogenetics and his wife. Daniel is painfully thin and gentle. He wrings his hands, he offers me cigarettes, more sugar, a chair, a footstool. I am very calm, very precise.

"Do I have a Mongoloid baby? Is he blind? Deaf? Left-handed? Green-eyed? *What is it?*"

"Well, we don't really know if it's anything at all. Why don't you wait until Aaron sees you on Friday?"

"Because I'm five and a half months pregnant and it's only Wednesday. Can't someone else draw the blood?"

"Dear lady, don't worry. Worrying won't help anything."

"Why can't you draw blood now? Why wait until Friday?"

Nothing is wrong. I'd know if something were really wrong.

Friday, August 26, 1977

Aaron draws blood. The possibility of a saline abortion fills me with terror. Why didn't they take our blood when they took my amniotic fluid? Aaron agrees with me. He tells me that he has argued for exactly such a procedure, but no one listens to him.

"Just this week," he tells me, "three women over thirty-five have given birth to Mongoloid children on this ward. It could have been avoided if they'd been tested."

Tonight we stay at Glenda's apartment in Jerusalem. It's quaint, perfect. She's left fresh bread, cheese, olives and coffee for us. She's off to visit her married lover. (All the married men seem to be having affairs. I don't know about the married women.)

No test results for five or six days. I can't sleep.

Child: Are you worried?

August 28, 1977

Rachael, your paternal grandmother, isn't here in Jerusalem. I *know* it's a "big" trip from Tel Aviv for someone without a car. I *know* she's taking care of five other people: her eldest daughter in the maternity hospital, her temporarily motherless grandson, her son-in-law. More: her own husband, who retired from work a year ago. Her youngest daughter, unmarried, who clings to her. *And still I want her to be with me.*

If we moved to Tel Aviv: next door, or around the corner, she'd rush in to us too, leave a cooked chicken, take a baby back with her. But I can't live in this noisy housing project. The frankness of the poverty—beds in living rooms, too few books, waiting lines for the toilet—returns me to my childhood. Which I flee still. To Jerusalem itself.

Rachael, Rachael: When will we see each other again? There is no ready-made home, no "set table" for me here with you.

You: who fled icy Europe for years of desert tents.

You: who are so cheerful, so loving.

You: whom your son misses. . . .

Lovely Lady: who laughed two years ago, after I explained feminism to you. "Good, but Mission Impossible," you said, holding me close.

*A*ugust 30, 1977

The founders of a feminist health collective in the Galil have come to Jerusalem to see me.

"We got together when we, as wives of faculty members, and as faculty ourselves, began having babies. The obstetrical care is horrendous. Unbelievable. No privacy, no pain-killers, a few ignorant midwives, filthy toilets, supercilious physicians, and pathetically frightened female patients."

"We want someone to hold each woman's hand when she's in labor. We want Arabic as well as Hebrew spoken. We want toilet paper, educated midwives, *human* doctors, and anesthetics as well as prepared natural childbirth. What do you think?"

Risa and Jean are long-time American-Jewish immigrants. They're vibrant, strong-willed. I tell them I'm waiting for blood test results and they grow silent with concern.

"Do you want to stay with us? The mountains are wet and mystical. Come, come back with us."

September 1, 1977

It's nothing! Nothing! Nothing! All three of us have these giant satellite cells. A family trait. Three large, harmless dancing bears in our genetic galaxy.

Never have I felt so sick. For three weeks my body has been traumatized. I've been to two laboratories, three doctors, and the hospital three times. Until today I assumed I had hepatitis, mononucleosis *and* dysentery.

And what, exactly, do I have? A gastrointestinal virus, exacerbated by my taking iron pills to combat the anemia of pregnancy.

September 7, 1977

"Ah, Phyllis, you're lucky to be pregnant. You agree, don't you, that a woman, especially a creative woman, *should* be a mother?"

"Ilana, I'm not sure. In fact, I feel so much at the mercy of my body, that I wonder whether the whole thing is possible."

"You know, Phyllis, my husband doesn't sleep with me. But I can't seem to leave him. I yearn for a baby. For each of us, there is some startling misfortune, some paralysis, some sorrow we live with, always. . . . The man who publishes my stories told me that a serious writer is too aggressive to be a mother. Do you think he's right?"

Ilana is my age. She is one of Jerusalem's "magic people": Talmudically moral, elegantly social. We walk, arm in arm. We stop for coffee every hour. We keep talking, reaching for ourselves through each other.

"Ilana," I finally say, "take a lover, become pregnant. You can stay with your husband. *Do it,* if you yearn for it so much."

But this is a land of grieving widows, of mothers struggling alone with fatherless children, of mothers who have lost son after son, daughter after daughter, to military death. The people here turn away from the sight of such unbearable sorrow. What am I telling her to do? How dare any woman influence, too powerfully, any other woman in her decision to have or not to have a child? I cannot interfere in another woman's dialogue with Life and Death.

The silence of mothers on the subject of motherhood when a non-mother is present. What unconsciously exquisite restraint. What a dangerous silence. How dare one's own mother be so thoughtlessly noisy, so powerfully insistent about this choice?

"Ilana, becoming a mother, like anything important, must demand some dangerous sacrifice. I'm not Superwoman. I don't know how well I'll be able to manage it. I'm frightened."

I don't want to leave Ilana. I'd like her to live near us, little one. I'd like Eva and Hava and Ada and Rachael, your grandmother, to live near us.

And soon, very soon, we're leaving them. We go back as we came: the three of us. Women, not even grandmothers, not even soul-mates, leave their own countries, their own families, to follow strange women into foreign lands.

Ruth and Naomi are storybook figures, engraved only on the heart of longing.

September 11, 1977

Back! Too much to do: see Frédéric, meet the midwife, buy some comfortable bras, shoes; interview students; confirm lectures; meet with my publisher; fly to Chicago—unpack! And that's just this week.

Oh, the advice you get when you're pregnant! Some women tell me to walk as much as possible. Others insist that elevating my feet and remaining in bed will do me the most good. Some women insist I avoid all salt, alcohol, sleeping pills. Some mothers warn me that my weight gain is dangerous—to you.

Everyone believes that whatever I do, feel, think, affects you totally. *They tell me to avoid all stress and anguish.* To "be happy." I'd better stop breathing altogether. They'd better put me into suspended animation. Someone had better give me the address of the Home for Pregnant Women—and get someone else to impersonate me so I don't renege on any of my commitments.

If I brood too much—about my pregnancy, about money, about the female condition—then it's assumed that this could cause your death.

What if it's true? What if that month of sleeping pills I took has already done you some great damage? What if those glasses of wine and all those anxious moments have already doomed you in some small and terrible way?

If anyone thinks pregnant women are entitled to loving care and careful feeding, then let them step forth now and provide it—or forever hold their peace. It is beyond my capacity to provide myself with the suggested amount of repose. Is there that much repose in the world? If there is, how do I know that *that's* what you need?

September 14, 1977

For a week now: no heartburn, no shortness of breath. "I" am not here anymore!

I don't inhabit my body any longer. My consciousness merely hovers nearby, unneeded for Nature's work. "I" am not my rising stomach, my weight gain, my swelling feet. "I" remain unchanged.

But everything is changing. Sometimes I move through the flow of my days like a great vessel through warm waters, buoyed up by the seas, nowhere near the ordinary shore. (Is this why formerly pregnant women have begun to look at me so wistfully, so nostalgically?)

September 19, 1977

Chicago. Today I was interviewed on television. The nearly all-female audience thrilled and embarrassed me by wanting to know more about my pregnancy than about my ideas or books.

One woman asked me if "this" meant I wouldn't write any more books.

"Do you think that 'working' mothers should work at motherhood only?" I ask her.

She did. This belief frightens me. So many women have sacrificed themselves to it. So many women feel that all mothers must do the same.

Why *have* a child, the Mothers say, if you're not there every moment to guard him against danger and to enjoy him while he's still young?

Why indeed? But can a child be a full-time occupation for a grown adult? For *all* grown adults? Maybe I'm suited only for four-hour-a-day child-guard duty and not for the grand round-the-clock shift.

How much power this belief has: that a child needs its natural mother for every day of five years—and that mothers who disappear for more than an hour a day are "unnatural" women, are *army deserters,* who deserve to be court-martialed by female opinion, who deserve to be shot for anything that goes "wrong" with their children.

Men march to *their* wars this way too: strait-jacketed by the deep and powerful beliefs of other men, filled with their own heady longings.

Doesn't anyone here realize that most mothers throughout history have always worked "inside" and "outside" the home?

Doesn't anyone remember grandmothers, older children, "helping" busy mothers with children? Doesn't anyone here want to talk about our long human history of hired wet nurses, governesses, housekeepers; our history of slave mothers for children?

Doesn't anyone here in this audience want to discuss the much-admired first ladies of Hollywood and Washington and their retinues of baby nurses, governesses, cooks, tutors, masseuses, chauffeurs—who turn America's female stars into "absentee" mothers?

No. No one really wants to.

"Good luck! Have an easy labor! Enjoy the baby!" the Mothers tell me on television.

September 21, 1977

The men at my university are displeased. My belly, my brain, offend their flatness. They will not forgive me for offending them. They have "doctored" my teaching schedule. Now I must leave home at 3 P.M. on Mondays, Tuesdays and Thursdays, and return close to midnight. Dusk-through-evening classes: the worst hours for me.

Why is everything I arranged so carefully with my chairman, Alan, turned upside down? Why have I been ordered to teach at precisely those hours when pregnant women grow drowsy, cranky? At precisely those hours I ruled out beforehand, for these reasons?

They're punishing me for daring to get pregnant—*by not treating me in a humane way.* The absence of child care at this university is logical. No parents or children are wanted.

No. I exaggerate. I see misogyny, conspiracies, where none exist. It's the frozen budget. It's Kafka's bureaucracy. Probably, *I* haven't gone about matters the right way. (Fill in the rest. You've heard it all. You even believe it a little.)

Why, then, does something nasty happen to so many women on the road to economic security—in universities and everywhere else?

Why was my friend Blanche, a full professor, scandalously fired by her university just as she lay anesthetized upon the table, having a Caesarean delivery?

Why was my overly qualified friend Julia kept out of a tenure-bearing line for ten years because she committed the sin of being a mother and a "faculty wife"? Why wasn't she hired "for real" by her department when her husband left her? When her husband wouldn't pay child support?

Why was my friend Edith forced to look for work in another state—and to leave the academic world entirely—when the demands of her motherhood were deemed "inappropriate" by her department?

Why are so many women never hired, hired last, paid least, fired first, because they are, or might become, mothers? Why are so many women treated this same way when it's suspected they won't ever become mothers?

This fact is so demonic that we find it easier to deny its existence; blame ourselves; decide "the job isn't worth it anyway." Not me. I know what they're doing—and why. *And I still can't believe it.*

I am "gross." They wish to "flatten" me.

September 24, 1977

Dinner with three "older" mothers: Miriam, Anna and Blanche. Miriam has four children between the ages of fifteen and twenty-five, and has produced four plays; Anna has two teen-aged sons and is a painter; Blanche has two children under ten and a Ph.D. What privileged, extraordinary women I know! How difficult their lives are: each still in search of a room of her own, and enough love and money to keep her going.

"Let's make a baby shower," they say, cynically, lovingly. I protest, but I glow.

A party, little one, a party with foolish furry animals; a party to herald your coming.

September 27, 1977

Frédéric wants to examine me every two weeks in October, and *every* week in November and December. He wants me to take a fetal heart monitoring test every month, starting right away. He wants a *twenty-four hour* urine sample collected twice a month, and two more ultrasound tests. He wants me to spend one hour every day lying on my left side and counting your kicks!

This is ridiculous! I'm being treated like I'm very ill, or dying. Doctors' visits, on this scale, are like forced childhood visits to pediatricians, to "specialists." The Long March of Childhood: not over yet. How can I take all these tests and keep my teaching and lecturing schedule? I've got to find a natural childbirth teacher, a midwife, a baby nurse.

Do I have to start choosing before you're born? Or do I choose to do everything—and collapse trying?

September 28, 1977

Becoming sensitive to *your* vulnerability, child, demands, as nothing else ever has, that I grow protective of my own vulnerability. Finally. Finally.

Over tea, I mention to Julia my awareness of violence.

"I'm feeling exposed, endangered, as my pregnancy progresses," I tell her. "People seem either indifferent or dangerous to me. City streets, *unkind remarks,* make me feel I need a cave to hide in."

"One does grow more sensitive to violence, to a human lack of sensitivity, to slights, upon becoming a mother."

"Julia: writing what I've written, why am I still so shocked that life isn't cherished? That people fear and kill what they love? In themselves and in others?"

We talk about fathers. We agree that real paternal involvement in child care will create a psychological revolution. I wonder what will happen once you've arrived: what will your father really do?

"Julia, tell me about your motherhood, about how you managed it all." Julia is in her fifties and has a twenty-year-old son.

"Well. I became pregnant a long time ago, when I was in my mid thirties. Twenty years ago that was an uncommon age to begin motherhood. Of course, I had household help. And university teaching is never full time. . . . I guess I slowed down on administration, on research, on writing. But a child is worth it." She beams at me.

"My son is my greatest friend."

September 30, 1977

Vera, of the marvelous, throaty voice and soothing manner, has cooked for me. Vera has two grown daughters. We talk about them—and about me.

"Once, Phyllis—don't judge by this tiny apartment—I led a different life: two large homes, all kinds of help with the children, plenty of time to indulge my desire to make money, to do volunteer work, to look good. It changed when I got divorced. Then the three of us lived right here, all together, on top of each other. And I worked at any job that would support us. . . . Eat, you're not eating," she reminds me. "But things have a way of working out. They really do. My girls are so special. Do you know, we all live in this building, in separate apartments!"

"Ah, Vera, I've never been so depressed before. Maybe I made a mistake. David can't earn very much money. The burden's too heavy."

"You know," she says calmly, "there are ups and downs in pregnancy. Don't be frightened by them. You wouldn't be pregnant if you didn't want to. You were serious enough about it to let your body act out your desire."

"Yes, that's true. But everything seems to be closing down, not opening up. I have no job offers, no real excitement about my new book—nothing but delays and silences. They humiliate me at school, and don't pay that well. There's no *communitas* in New York. There's only dinners for two—like this lovely one—and then back to one's own struggle for survival. I'm lonely. I've never been so lonely before."

"Let me give you some stones to rub between your fingers. They'll soothe you. Come, choose some."

I pick three smooth, pretty stones to keep. I want to hide how depressed I really am. She can't understand how blue, how very blue I am. Why burden her?

"Phyllis, why don't we listen to some women sing the

blues? I have a fine collection. Here, sit down and sing along. I know you used to be a singer."

Music! Music helps. At midnight, I'll be thirty-seven. My last birthday without you. Suddenly I miss your father. I want his chest, the crook of his arm, to fall asleep in.

Good night, Dinah Washington, Billie Holiday, Bessie Smith, Sarah Vaughan, Peggy Lee, Ella Fitzgerald. Good night, Vera. And thank you all.

October 1, 1977

What depression, irritability, seize me. I feel so cramped: my liver, my gut, squeezed out of shape by you, expanding.

I spent this morning with seventeen-year-old Nancy, who spoke so quietly I could hardly hear her. Nancy: raped last night. Nancy: whose mother couldn't prevent this.

Child: The task requires too much unending courage. Once, I worked with a woman whose daughter became fatally ill when she was five years old. We never discussed it. What if everyone flees our tragedies too?

Hamburgers, and late-afternoon wine.

"Meg, I'm afraid of what I've done. Don't say 'I told you so.' It's too late for that."

"Phyllis, you're tough. It'll work out. If it doesn't, well, many of our dreams don't. . . . "

"This is not a dream. It's what really flies out of Pandora's Box."

"Well, it's a tough time for all us dreamers. There's a lot of bills to pay—especially when you're broke. I've always said you should live more thriftily. Pay as little rent as possible. Move to a smaller place."

"With a baby coming?"

Dusk in SoHo. She doesn't understand what I feel—but then neither do I. Not totally.

October 9, 1977

I dream a wonderful dream. I give birth to a little blond boy. We fall into conversation immediately in the white-tiled delivery room. He laughs uproariously. He is very small, but gets bigger as we talk. He tells me that his name is "Alyce" or "Alan," and begins to talk to me about books!

I wake up suffused with pleasure and excitement. I remember his face exactly. Is it your face? Have you really visited me in a dream? Are you requesting a name that begins with an *A*?

October 12, 1977

When I was lecturing in Ohio today, one professor stood up and said: "Dr. Chesler, here you are, obviously pregnant. Could you please make some comment on this fact?" She thinks my being pregnant somehow repudiates either my feminism or my doctorate. Possibly both. She thinks my body is more important than the "ideas" I have. She thinks my body somehow negates my ability to have ideas.

"Well," I say, "you don't really know how I got pregnant. As a matter of fact, it was a Goddess who made me pregnant. I'm one woman in a long line, Leda, the Virgin Mary, who've been visited from afar . . ."

After the laughter, the annoyance, died down, I talked about the importance of not automatically assuming *anything* about a woman's pregnancy.

My body is a statement that requires further explanation. Confinement/exposure. They are the same.

October 15, 1977

One of my two brothers is getting married. *This* is my mother's main concern. She calls daily to share her thoughts about caterers, photographers, dance bands.

She calls *to be listened to.* As if she's the daughter and I the mother! As if my swelling belly is less important than a wedding—or too important to discuss.

Is this impending grandmotherhood traumatic for her? Is this thing that she desires so difficult for her? *Does she really desire my motherhood?*

October 22, 1977

Today, as I was lecturing in Boston, a mother with two children under ten stood up and asked me how to bring up children in a non-sexist way! So deeply ingrained is the female distrust of our own experience and perceptions!

"I'm not even a mother yet," I told her. "You're already an expert—certainly an expert in your own children. What could *I* possibly tell you that you don't know? I may be an author, but I've never fed an infant. I've never stayed up all night worrying about a baby. I've never comparison-shopped for play groups, baby-sitters, part-time jobs or pediatricians. *And I'm scared I can't do it.*"

Afterward, dinner with Rita, my former colleague and friend, who is separated and mother to an eight-year-old daughter. Rita patiently answers my questions.

"I was depressed for five years after Marcy was born. I don't know if it was the marriage, my job, or the sheer fatigue of child care. Now things are better. Her father still keeps trying to get custody, but settles for very good visitation rights."

"Who takes care of Marcy and the house while you're at work?"

"I have a very lucky arrangement. My house is big enough to offer a couple with a baby their own space, in return for Marcy's mothering and house care. If I didn't have them, I suppose I'd kill myself."

"How did you find this miracle couple?"

"By advertising."

I decide to start an ad campaign. (Where? What should I advertise for: a wife? a mother?)

October 24, 1977

Margaret Mead paid me a visit today. In January we had met each other in public dialogue in Cincinnati. We talked of many things privately, including my desire to become pregnant. She'd hugged me goodbye, told me to come to her when I was pregnant. A woman of my word, I called her a month ago.

Now she's insisted on coming to see me, because "being pregnant is more fragile a state than being old." As she comes in, removing her cape, positioning her walking stick, her first question, before we sit down, is: "What are you doing about your nipples?" This is something my own mother hasn't asked. I say: "Nothing."

"Rub them with a rough washcloth, pinch them, toughen them up," she tells me. Bluntly. Simply.

I ply her with questions about organization and management: "How do you keep breast-feeding when you have public lectures to give?"

"Take a nursemaid and the baby with you wherever you go. That's what I did when Catherine was born."

I'm listening intently for all the advice I can get. Mead looks around at my crowded apartment.

"Try not to work at home. Get an office outside and try to find a woman with a child who needs shelter, because you can provide that and *she* can provide you with mothering—and a child companion for a baby. You'll have to move to larger quarters, of course."

Of course.

"And don't listen to anyone—I don't care if he's a doctor or your best friend—who discourages breast-feeding."

We talk about the problems that arise when a "professional" woman becomes a mother "late in life." As she did at thirty-eight. As I'm doing at thirty-seven. "What happens is significant and incredibly joyful," she assures me, "if you have your work and enough money."

Of course.

I admire her crustiness, her grandiosity, the fact that she's survived, triumphed. How lucky I am that such a visible grandmother of our American tribe came to see me about you. Clearly, she takes initiation of women into motherhood seriously.

October 25, 1977

I want an "older" woman for midwife. Someone who attended my mother at my birth. A sacred connection.

My mother didn't have a midwife. Frédéric introduces me to Shifra, the only nurse-midwife in the hospital.

"You're the first private patient who's wanted a midwife," she says.

She's cold. "No-nonsense" is the term. She takes my medical history. (I'm always afraid I'll leave out some vital information that can save my life.) She's at least five feet ten. I follow her to an examining room.

Legs spread, socks on, it's a different atmosphere with her than with the kindest male doctor. There is no shame. No pretended indifference.

Fingers in, hand pushing down on my belly. "You're hurting me," I tell her. Resentfully.

"That's O.K. You have good pelvic bones. I want to see you every other week."

Another appointment.

"Will you be with me from the beginning to the end?" I ask. Shyly. Only a girl-child would still want her Mommy with her when she gives birth—or dies. This setting—stirrups and busy loudspeakers—is "above," against, such a tiny human request.

"Depends on who else needs me and what stage you're in," she answers. "Depends on how long it takes me to drive into the city. Depends on the weather, the traffic. Depends on whether I'm reachable when you call."

"Would you consider coming to my house and staying with me until we absolutely have to go to the hospital?" I ask. Embarrassed. Fearful.

"That's Frédéric's decision. He's the one who arranged to get me on the private ward."

"What I want is a private midwife arrangement." I try again.

"Let's see how it proceeds," she says, washing her hands, looking at her watch.

Why don't I just deliver at home with a midwife in attendance? With a physician on call? Because I don't know any physician who'll do it. Because I can't stop my life to search for one. Because I want Frédéric.

Because I'm afraid. If enough women supported me, with personal experience, with specific information about home birth, I'd probably do it that way. But I know so few pregnant women, so few new mothers to give me names of private midwives. I know *no one.*

October 26, 1977

Lecturing in Toronto, I pace. I declaim. The videotape camera follows me. After two hours I'm flushed, faint.

"The lights are too hot," I call out. "I need a chair, please."

"But that'll ruin the tape," the technicians tell me.

"I'm a little nauseous," I say.

"Don't sit," a woman in the audience protests. "We can hear you better if you keep standing."

Where, now, the courtesies for pregnant women? The opened doors, the proffered seats? Or do you renounce all that by taking a public role? Am I supposed to pretend I'm *not* pregnant? Is it poor form for a feminist to *be* pregnant? Or is it taboo to be on stage as an authority, and pregnant too?

October 28, 1977

I've just called all the housekeeper–baby nurse agencies. Today, I interview ten women. No one really wants the job of "wife" to another woman. Feeding the baby—yes. Feeding the baby's father—no. The baby's laundry—yes. The laundry of the baby's mother—no. Light shopping sometimes—yes. But someone else would have to watch the baby. Cleaning—never. Ironing—out of the question.

On the open market, a *staff* is required to perform the work of one overworked wife and mother. A butler to answer the door, accept deliveries. A cook to cook. A lady's maid for sewing, ironing and laundry. A cleaning woman to clean. (Everything but windows. No windows.) An errand runner to pick up forgotten milk, fresh bread, emergency prescriptions. *Three* child care specialists to do nothing but watch the child in eight-hour shifts for twenty-four hours, seven days a week.

Who can afford a staff? What kind of person will I end up settling for—gratefully? How long will she stay?

How can I live with two strangers—you and your nurse? Who but the wealthiest of women can pay for a housekeeper *and* a child care person? Who but the wealthiest New Yorker has enough space so that privacy exists even after childbirth?

Where will I write if not at home?

November 1, 1977

I'm obsessed with wallpapering the apartment. I've been to three wallpaper stores. I choose twenty samples. I just bought ten plants. If I settle them all in one window, we can open a health food restaurant.

No two dishes are alike. The salad bowl has been cracked for years. I have no matching silverware, no candlesticks.

Why am I suddenly aware of all this? Do I want to impress you, child, with a buffet dinner by candlelight?

Child: Your mother and father live like bachelors. We mainly eat out. When we eat in, we eat standing up. We never entertain. Your coming from so far away embarrasses me into emotions of hospitality. What can I do to make you feel at home?

The kitchen (!) is not quite six feet long, five feet wide. There's room for one person, standing. It's as drab-dark in there as a Russian winter courtyard in late afternoon.

I can't live in such cramped quarters. You're squeezing me: lungs, gut, kidney. I need room to expand. I want to give you a "baby's" room. Yellow. Purple. White. I want to sit there in a rocking chair, my hair in a single braid, singing.

I'll call everyone I know about secondhand baby furniture. (What? Nothing new?) Already I'm a bad mother. There's too much to do. And there's no baby yet.

November 7, 1977

A surprise party for me—the mother!—at Nora's. Carolyn, Sharon, Joan and Meg: all there. Nora's cooking: soup with basil, a seafood platter with butter sauce, a homemade mousse pie, dark coffee.

We talk politics: a mysteriously destroyed printing press, an abortion clinic closed-down, the Equal Rights Amendment.

This family of friends: how careful we are not to presume too much. None of us exposes her starving child to the others.

We have each been attacked, daily, by that starving child let loose in other women. We will share our dreams and take our starving children elsewhere: into battle, into work.

Carolyn gives me two precious stones—amazonite—for beauty, for strength during labor. From Sharon: a cream satin nightgown.

"I see you in flowing garments," she says.

A burgundy shawl from Nora to warm myself in during labor, and at home when I wander about afterward. She's pinned a now defunct "Sisterhood Is Powerful" button on it.

Joan gives me lovely Japanese women, painted on coasters.

Meg unfurls a huge line painting she's done of me, pregnant. She calls it "An Imaginary Portrait of Phyllis During the Great Pregnancy."

All the gifts are for me: the mother-to-be. The greatest gift is these women, themselves, this evening. They honor me by the way they lead their lives.

Ah! For the respect and friendship of such women I would do anything. I have.

November 9, 1977

I've found a private natural childbirth teacher, a mother of three, who lives six blocks away. Her name is April. Her bathroom carpet, wallpaper, towels, all match.

Her first lecture—with illustrations—on fetal development and childbirth is fascinating. Why hasn't anyone told me any of this before? Why isn't the birth process routinely pondered, praised, everywhere? Is this universal fact of human origin an exclusive secret: one that only pregnant women in prepared-childbirth classes get to discuss? Is pregnancy still a tale told to medical specialists only, and not to the rest of us, male and female, pregnant and non-pregnant?

April has a naked rubber doll for demonstration purposes. I want to play with it. I want to stuff it in my vagina and pull it out. I want to walk out leaving it behind. I want to take it home with me.

November 12, 1977

My mother hisses at me, minces for her sons. (Four years ago, I asked her to help me type a manuscript to meet a deadline. Reluctantly she agreed. And came five hours late. "I was doing your brother's laundry.")

Now she's called me *eleven* times on the phone to remind me that tonight there's a pre-wedding dinner for my brother.

I go. The cigarette smoke overwhelms me. After a half hour I'm nauseous and have a headache. She doesn't notice. After an hour and a half I have to leave.

"Don't carry on," she says. "You're not the first woman to be pregnant. If smoke bothers you, how can you fly everywhere to lecture?"

She indulges your two uncles. Never me. Not even when I'm pregnant with you, her first grandchild. I am robbed of my Mother's kisses. I am inconsolable.

Flushed, feverish. I can't sleep. Your father watches me. Why doesn't he kill them for me—my insensitive, "fragile" brothers; my mother, *their* indulgent servant?

"Phyllis," he says gently, "your mother had to treat you as someone special—someone not like her—for a long time. She can't impose on you, the way others impose on her. Now you're pregnant. She'll be damned if she treats you 'specially.' Now that you really need it—in her terms. Anyway, Superwoman doesn't need a mother to rescue her from cigarette smoke, or to hold her hand."

Oh, but she does. I do.

November 14, 1977

Shifra examines me on the ward. She shows me the "natural childbirth" room: an ordinary hospital room with a small purple throw rug on the floor and colored curtains at the window. I look out at the park across the street. The park I walked in when I worked here, went to medical school here.

Women are screaming on either side of me. Across the hall too.

"Please come in. Somebody. Help me. I'm dying."

I run into the hallway. I see two nurses pass the room of screams. One makes a face.

"Why don't you go in to her?" I ask one of them.

"Look, honey. We're busy. She won't remember any of this. She's in a very advanced stage of labor. We can't do anything for her now anyway."

"You can *be* with her," I say.

"Maybe *you're* a little too sensitive yourself." The nurse walks off, wheels around. "Don't you go messing in there."

I stand at the doorway. That woman, covered with a sheet, is a young girl. The setting turns her into a monster. Wild-eyed with fear. In pain. I freeze. My human impulses are shamed, silenced by everyone else's indifference.

One woman is having a miscarriage. Another is in the painful throes of a saline abortion. A woman is screaming in Spanish: an operatic solo to the Mother of God. *"Madre de Dios,"* she implores, she trills.

"That woman is doing her thing," the nurse tells me.

November 20, 1977

The leg cramps! They seize me by night. I leap straight up into the air out of sleep, shrieking. This is the only pain I fear: a leg cramp.

Your father always wakes up. He massages my calf. He orders me to flex my foot. I'm terrorized by pain.

What do athletes do? Can you ever get used to this kind of pain?

What if labor is like this? I'll lose heart. I'll become a desperate child. I'll beg for drugs.

Maybe I should find a hypnotist.

No. I want to be there with you.

November 22, 1977

"Come, be with me while I'm still single," I tease my comrade in literary arms, Grace. "Once I give birth, I'm married—to the baby."

"Oh, Phyllis, I'm very busy, very committed. To more important things."

Grace—Grace!—won't visit me. We have loved each other for seven years. I miss her deeply. My choice to become pregnant is not "important": reduces *me* to non-importance.

Would I visit a pregnant woman every week "just" because she was pregnant? Have I ever?

November 24, 1977

Today my brother got married. Afterward I fought with my mother.

She didn't want to come home with me. She'd made a "prior plan." I am flooded with emptiness. My mother's not comfortable with me. (I'm not comfortable with her.) She's so terrified of being rejected by me (and I by her) that she rejects first. (She must be angrier than I am.) She denies herself what she wants. (Does she want anything with me? What?) (Me.) Unlike me, she thinks to avoid suffering. She doesn't go looking for "trouble." She never expects anything from anyone. I do—and am always disappointed. By Her.

My mother will "hate" me as long as I'm not like her. As long as I expect her to mother me. Can I ever forgive her for not loving me for my strength? What strength?

I'll have to. But how?

Bitter legacy.

November 29, 1977

I sit on the hospital bed, a thick belt strapped across my abdomen. It's connected to a squat machine. Your heartbeat accelerates whenever you move. And gets recorded on the machine's ticker tape.

What if you're sleeping? What if you don't want to be recorded?

Move, baby. Move for Mama. I want to get out of here with proof that you're normal. Ah, there you go, rolling over, my little sea wave.

Things you know about me: The red cave of my uterus. The taste of my bloodstream. The sound of me, inhaling oxygen.

No one else knows this about me. Not even myself.

I go over my final list with Frédéric. My conditions: that your father room in; that I'm not put into stirrups or strapped down in any way; that I hold you and breast-feed you before they clean you up or inject silver nitrate into your eyes; that no internal fetal heart monitor be used; that I'm not tied down to an intravenous; that an episiotomy be avoided if possible; that I be shaved very minimally; that your father be allowed to stay during a Caesarean if one is needed.

The more I demand, the more I have to smile. The more "reasonable" and diplomatic I have to be. I can't show my feelings or fears ("strident, hysterical"). I can't issue orders ("pushy, aggressive").

Pregnancy is no reprieve from being treated like a womb-man.

December 2, 1977

Early morning. In bed, watching you: flesh-bumps, flesh-jumps, abdomen-bubbles, small belly-quakes. With all your might, you appear—dancing! Sporting with me: cooking-bubbles, flesh-walks. What amazing pleasure!

Late afternoon: I must have a breadbox. A place to store the loaf after it's baked. I'm off on a Hero's journey. No one sells breadboxes anymore. Unexpectedly, I meet Nora in the domestics section of Gimbels East. She's in search of an electric broom.

What can this mean? we ask, laughing. There are men at meetings *now*, this very minute, figuring out how to blow up the planet . . . and here we are, trying to spruce it up, keep it clean. *Here we are,* in Domestics! Does this have any larger meaning?

Evening: I give a lecture in New Jersey. Half the women claim having a child is more wonderful than anything else. The other half claim that it ruined their lives.

December 3, 1977

A bad dream: I gave birth to a teen-age daughter. We fight. She doesn't like me. She leaves me in the delivery room! I wake up devastated. Does this mean I'm a woman-hater??? The dream with the little blond boy was so different. . . .

Is that me, leaving my mother?

Is that my own daughter self leaving, to be replaced by a mother self? Why is my daughter angry with me? Why am I so hurt?

Must she go?

December 5, 1977

Frédéric just told me he's leaving for Switzerland. He said it casually, just as I was leaving his office. He'll be away until December 23. I walk alone in the heavy rain for an hour. Stung. Furious.

How dare he leave me now?

What if I go into labor while he's away? What then? He's given me the name of a stranger who "covers" for him. I'd rather deliver myself at home, alone.

How can he leave me now?

December 10, 1977

No one but me seems to notice how slow I am. How difficult each thing is for me to do. No one but me is bothered by this.

In colors of blood and air I spin without stopping: colon, foot, eye. By day, by night, for nine months, I weave you: precisely. Faithfully. No wonder I'm slow at other tasks.

What do we spin today? The shape of your smile? A last-minute gesture? Do we go over, once more, what's already there? Checking up, making sure that nothing's been forgotten?

Ah! You're moving through the eons, the centuries, more swiftly now, growing larger. The design grows thicker, swings back and forth on the loom of me. Testing it. Making sure it will hold. Making sure it will break.

I wish I could see you! I wish I could play with you, just once, while you're still in me.

You'd frighten me. I'd be a tiny visitor, shipwrecked, disturbing your great sleep. Would you look at me with one red eye? Crush me by turning over? Devour me, spit out my bones? What would you sound like?

Are you lonely?

December 15, 1977

"Please," I say, "let me teach part-time in the spring. Or full time, but based somewhere in Manhattan. I plan to breast-feed. It'll be impossible to run back and forth from Manhattan to Westchester every two hours. It *takes* two hours round trip! The college doesn't have an infant nursery. I *do* want to teach. I have thirty students who definitely want to study with me at your Manhattan branch. . . ."

"Why don't you just make up your mind? Do you want to teach or be a mother?" the Administrator snarls at me.

"Do you actually mean what you're saying?" I ask.

"If you don't like it, bitch, why don't you quit?" his associate says.

We're standing in the cafeteria, surrounded by people. No one can hear us.

I visit my chairman.

"Alan, what should I do? What can I do?" I ask.

"Can you get out of this place?" he sighs. "Phyllis, I'd love for you to be able to teach part-time. I've brought it up three times. The administration and some of your colleagues—you can guess who—behave badly. It's their legal prerogative to refuse this request. I can bring it up again.

"There's something else." He hands me a memo to him from "above." Dated today. It's an order that Alan immediately "investigate" a student's complaint about me. *Another* complaint. This student claims that since I'm not giving a final examination—only a series of papers—that I *might* fail her, and she'd have no recourse.

"Every year I'm brought up on 'charges,'" I whisper. It's as if I have to justify my right to work. Over and over again. Being pregnant changes nothing. Publishing changes nothing. Makes it worse I think."

"I know they're trying to screw you out of your medical benefits," Alan whispers. "You'd better take some action."

"I'm so tired. . . ."

"Phyllis, go on sick leave immediately. You look like you'll give birth any day now. You can't afford to fight the bureaucracy forever," Alan says.

"The bureaucracy pays my rent. If I stop fighting back, I won't be resting. I'll be out looking for other money sources, or eating myself up alive, worrying about it."

Child: No one takes my need for money seriously. That possibility—that a pregnant woman leads a precarious economic life—is something both friends and strangers don't want to think about.

"She should have married for money—like I had to do."

"She must have made a fortune. Isn't she *famous?*"

"Don't *have* a baby, Phyllis, if you haven't figured out a way to beat the system. Your bed—lie in it. Quietly."

December 20, 1977

Child: I admit it. I'm afraid. What if the pain is unbearable? What if I'm treated cruelly when I'm too helpless to defend myself?

What if you're born monstrous: with my anger, my excesses?

What if you're stillborn?

What if you're killed by some hospital procedure?

Should I heat cauldron water, cut your cord with my bloody teeth?

I have no one to talk to about this. Women's smiles are fixed grins: the grimace of masks, of silence. I know they smell my fear, want not to remember their own. They keep their distance. Only your father hugs me, holds me close.

December 24, 1977

Will you come tonight? Will you? The moon, fat and orange, tells me: "No."

I'm moon-struck. I dance alone in Central Park. Look: the trees are wearing light bulbs. New Yorkers are smiling at each other. Something unnatural is afoot.

The birth of a child in winter, when earth sleeps, when Woman brings forth fruit even when Nature can't. The human miracle. Northern style.

December 30, 1977

You're still in me. I'm still in you. There's no more room. Why won't you let go of me?

Look at me: huge, irritable, on the phone. Can I teach my courses in Manhattan? No. Can I bring a grievance case against the college for fouling up my medical plan? No. I'm on hold with the health insurance bureaucracy for hours.

Hurry, baby, get me off the phone.

The mail piles up, like the snow outside, menacingly white. What if the cars can't move? Will they take me to the hospital by sled?

Are you coming? Have you changed your mind?

December 31, 1977

I—and fifty thousand others—have the flu. It's urban malaria. Nothing "serious." I just can't move or think or swallow. I can't breathe at all.

How will I deep-breathe for natural childbirth?

Time is stuck. If you don't come out this week, I'm forgetting the whole thing.

Part Two

CHILDBIRTH

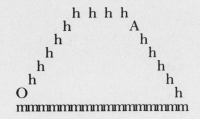

8:30 P.M. It's you! You've begun. I'm giddy. Positively light-headed. I'd better be: tonight I oppose myself into motherhood.

Tonight I descend, tonight I rise. Tonight I am halved, tonight I am doubled. Tonight I lose you forever, tonight I meet you for the first time. Tonight I cheat death. Tonight I die.

Palpable, luminous, the Mysteries unfold: arcs of paradox. I can touch them. I am them.

Time	*Length of Contraction*
8:35 P.M.	68 seconds
8:42 P.M.	52 seconds
8:47 P.M.	61 seconds

Child: You've had your last bloody meal. Soon I'll turn red milk white. The most natural miracle of all.

Little Theseus: I've thrown you the golden double-helix. You've followed it as far as it will go. We're alone now. Soon, soon, you'll appear at my threshold, hungry, shipwrecked. As all Heroes do.

I sprinkle some wine on the floor. For luck. Farewell! Bon voyage! Will we meet before dawn? That unearthly hour when Earth slows down, ever so slightly, for the arrival of new souls?

9:12   9:16   9:22   9:28   9:32   9:40   9:45

We've been traveling to meet each other for both our lifetimes. For three weeks you've been sending messengers of brownish mucus. For ten days my cervix has softened for you, opened two centimeters for you. I'm ready to receive you, little one.

   10:14   10:18   10:24   10:31   10:39   10:43

Will you suddenly tumble out? Can this happen? I'd better call the midwife.

"Hello, Shifra?" I say. "I'm having sixty-second contractions every four to eight minutes. For two hours now."

                10:59   11:04   11:07

"Try to sleep, Phyllis," she tells me. "It sounds like prodromal labor."

"What's that?" *How many more words are there, mysterious to me, to describe what I'm going to do?*

"I'm having one right now. . . ."

                11:11   11:16   11:21

"It'll go on for a while, without any significant dilation of the uterus. Save your strength for later on," she advises me.

"How can I sleep if each contraction hurts?"

"You'll be surprised what you can do. Sleep between contractions," she says.

I don't believe her. You're coming soon. Aren't you?

January 5, 1978

I time your movements with a stopwatch. I sip wine. It's past midnight. I sit in bed, propped against the wall. I have one whole page covered with the rhythm of your descent.

12:20   12:27   12:32   12:37   12:40

"Try to calm down," your father says. Then: "Can you try and sleep?" he asks.

"Are you crazy?" I exclaim. "Of course not."

Out in the living room, I dance with you. Don't worry: I won't drop you.

2:12 A.M.	57 seconds
2:17 A.M.	65 seconds
2:24 A.M.	58 seconds

My throat is flu-sore. My nose is stuffed. How will I do my breathing exercises if I can't breathe?

Back in bed. With both sets of fingertips I massage my belly, making double circles during each contraction. (It's called effleurage.) Can you feel me doing this? *The contractions hurt. You hurt. I hurt.* I'm doing the first breathing exercises. Maybe I'm starting it too soon?

3:10 A.M.	64 seconds
3:14 A.M.	58 seconds
3:19 A.M.	61 seconds

Oh! Into the grinning jaws of death I'd be walking were I a woman of another century. I remember the tombstones in Vermont, New Hampshire, Massachusetts. Grassy, lonesome.

4:40 A.M.	38 seconds
4:43 A.M.	56 seconds

"Beloved daughter of . . . First wife of . . . Dead in childbirth . . . Buried here with her dead child . . . with her female successor . . . with her survivor husband and surviving children."

5:23 A.M.	63 seconds
5:28 A.M.	56 seconds
5:33 A.M.	51 seconds

Those tiny, tiny tombstones over skeletons new-born in 1749 and 1862.

6:24 A.M.	52 seconds
6:29 A.M.	65 seconds
6:33 A.M.	59 seconds

It's light outside. I'm nauseous with fatigue. Ten hours and I'm still without you. (You're still with me.) All I have is a record of your movements. The world's unchanged.

7:40   7:46   7:51   7:59   8:04   8:09

Dozing. I wake to pain.

9:20   9:29   9:34   9:40   9:45

Time to call Frédéric.

"Finally!" he says. "Come in and let's examine you. Don't eat anything."

"Aren't you coming?" your father asks. "You're not even dressed."

10:38 A.M.	30 seconds
10:45 A.M.	42 seconds

"Why don't you go to Frédéric's without me?" I say. "I'm too tired. The baby's not moving very much. Maybe he's gone back to sleep. . . ."

Noon. Frédéric's office is filled with women in varying states of pregnancy. For once, I'm seen immediately.

"You're two and a half centimeters dilated, but you're not in active labor. I'd like to admit you to the hospital as soon as a bed is ready."

"Can I rest somewhere here?" I ask.

Frédéric kisses me on both cheeks and helps me up onto an examining table that's not in use. He dims the lights. I lie here, disappointed.

Your father slips in with a blood-red rose and forbidden candy. Courtship!

Exhaustion reduces me to slow motion. I can't think clearly. What should I do next? Take a walk? Return home? Why are we going to the hospital?

Outside. Walk back to the car. Get in. Sit. Drive to the hospital, up the ramp to the fifth parking level. Get out. Stand up. Cold. It's cold. Wait for the garage elevator. Descend to street level. I have to pee. Wait. Get inside the hospital first. Walk past the clinic benches to the elevator banks. Get in. I have to pee. Wait. The elevator is stopping at every floor. I get off at the sixth floor: "Labor and Delivery." Enter through the double swinging doors.

I notice everything. There are too many distractions: they slow me down. Time is slowing down.

1:00 P.M. I have come here to die. Why else would I be in a hospital? The ward seems deserted. No screams, no loudspeakers. Am I here alone? Your father helps me up onto the jack-knifed bed.

Where are you? Why aren't you moving?

Onto my right side, face the wall, for an enema. The nurse smiles. Growing flushed now. Into the bathroom. I exist: I can shit. All systems are functioning. Back up onto the bed.

1:40   1:45

There you are. You're moving again.

A smiling resident inserts a glucose intravenous into my left arm. Plastic snakes to my left, a sheer drop of wall to my right. Smiling strangers. Where am I?

"Why am I suddenly so sleepy?"

"Demerol in the glucose," your father whispers. "To take the edge off the contractions." *What contractions? There aren't any. How dare they drug me? Well, maybe I can rest for a while. Get some strength back. . . .*

Drifting. Where am I? Can you happen without me? I swim up into focus. *What time is it? What's happening?*

"You haven't dilated at all since Frédéric examined you three hours ago. It's three o'clock in the afternoon." Here's Shifra. In her nurse's uniform. *Oh. I'd hoped it would have happened while I rested. She's annoyed with me for being so slow.*

"I'll be here for good now, Phyllis," she says.

Surfacing. Frédéric comes in. "I'll stay in the hospital until you deliver. I've brought paperwork with me," he says. And disappears.

Wait. Am I giving birth or not?

"Do you want some oxytocin to speed things up?" Frédéric is back. "You've been up all night. The afternoon's nearly over. . . ."

"No. I don't want to lose control. I want it to happen by itself." *Liar! Tell him to drug you and be done with it.*

Something's sharp. Irritable. Is it me? "The Demerol's worn off," Shifra says. "Now we'll see some action." My throat is burning-sore. How will I be able to pant? I'm headachy with lack of sleep. *I have no strength. How will I deliver you?*

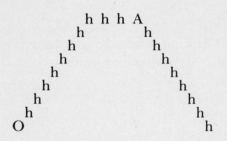

Can I get out of this?

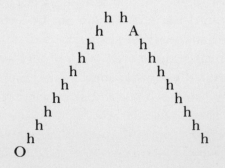

I'm cold with terror.

There's no turning back. I'm on my way to Venus, way past the moon, to bring you back. I breathe "properly" with each contraction. I don't dare not to.

What is this strange pain in, at, near my lower back? A low flame. Dull. Constant. It's back labor.

Your father kisses my face. He's up on the bed with me, ice-packing my back. Massaging it.

My eyes plead: stay don't ever leave me hold me help me go away. Leave me alone.

Time contracts. Thickens.

David (on tape, afterward): It took you two and a half hours to dilate to 5 centimeters. Then, at about 7 P.M. Frédéric and Shifra both agreed to give you Pitocin to speed things up.

No Pitocin! I'm deathly afraid of roller coasters.

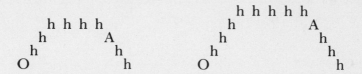

David: I could tell you were in a lot of pain. You didn't complain anymore. Your whole body tensed up during each contraction. You covered your face with your hand and put your face into the pillow. You didn't scream or cry. I hid my tears from you.

Something for my back. Please give me something.

David: You said you couldn't go through with it, that your back hurt constantly. Your teeth began to click. They stopped chattering when I kissed you, talked to you, washed your face. You grew cold. The contractions were longer, more frequent. I could tell when a contraction was beginning. From the fetal heart monitor machine. I told you: "O.K., one's about to begin. Here it comes." They were lasting between sixty and ninety seconds. When twenty seconds passed by, I'd say: "You're doing wonderfully. It's peaked already. It's nearly over." I tricked you psychologically.

*4/4 Breathing. Deep breathing. It works. It helps. But I'm so
alone. No one sees me. I can't hear anything.*

```
         h h h h h
      h            A              h h h h
   h            h             h            A
O              h          O              h h h h h h h
```

David: When a contraction ended I kissed you all over.
I told you how brave you were. I kept massaging your back.
With ice. With my hands.

*Something for my back. Something for my back. I can't stand
it. It's too bright in here. I can't see.*

Shifra: "She's ten centimeters dilated."

I am? Where are you, then?

Shifra: "O.K., Phyllis. You can start pushing. Right here
in bed."

January 6, 1978

Midnight. It's not working. *I'm* not working. I have no "overwhelming urge" to push. I want to give up, to give you up; to give birth. But I can't.

"Take the breath and hold it when the contraction starts," Shifra says. "Otherwise it's not effective."

Just give me a minute to rest. But you don't. You keep coming. There are so many pinpoints, all light-years away: galactic openings for you to enter through. I keep missing you. . . . What if I catch someone else?

Your longest journey is so short. How many inches must you actually cross over into being? Don't be frightened. Someday this journey will end. This journey never ends. I'm filled with pity and terror for you.

Which one of us is being born?

Gulliver is in childbirth, tied down by only one Lilliputian. I lie large, completely helpless. Now what, little one?

My tiny Jonah. My little trapped man-child, waiting to be spit out, whole. Your whale heaves. She's beached, exhausted.

David: Sometime after midnight, maybe one or two o'clock in the morning, you were transferred to the delivery room. A strange nurse put your feet into stirrups. I took them down. Then another nurse tied your legs to the stirrups. It left marks on you. I yelled at her. I untied you.

Too tired to say anything. I push with all my might. I'm the Lilliputian. I may not may not may not be able to do it. It's beyond me to give birth to you.

I am in labor, laboring. Moving through eons of sand. Walking the oceans. Looking for you. Beside myself with grief. Where are you hiding? Are you lost? Why do you linger?

David: Your back was hurting constantly. You had no more energy. Shifra was dozing. Frédéric was sleeping somewhere. I was trying to move you up and down myself. Helping you find a comfortable position. Massaging your back.

You're "sunny side up." Facing the top of my uterus. Pressing on my back with yours. That's why I'm in "back labor." I have to turn you around, slowly, before I can push you down. Twisting me round, slowly, as I rise, high above the crowd. *I'm so thirsty. Water. Please.*

Jerusalem silence. Time is absolutely still. I have been here forever. Time no longer exists. Always, time holds steady for birth. An eternal midwife. Time is irrelevant. There is only this rocketing, this labor.

I am absolutely alone. I watch from above, recording this terrible break with reality. *There are people down there, but I can't hear them very well.* If I must, I can speak through my body.

"My back."

"Water."

I hear my words return slowly, separately, back up to me.

David: You'd been pushing for nearly four hours. "We might have to do a Caesarean," Frédéric said. He left to get a second opinion. I saw your face. My heart stopped. You were giving up.

Shifra: "You can do it, Phyllis. I know you can."

Forgive me. Forgive me baby. I can't give birth to you.

David: Shifra heard "Caesarean" and really jumped up. She got another nurse. The three of us started to yell in chorus at you.

Shifra: "You can do it Mama. C'mon, take a deep breath close your mouth keep it closed hold that breath hold it hold it hold it hold it Now *PUSH PUSH PUSH PUSH PUSH PUSH PUSH KEEP THAT PUSH.*"

Me: I can hear you. Just barely. Yes.

David and Shifra: "Again. Breathe. Hold it. Hold it. Hold it. That's it. Now *PUSH GODDAMN IT PUSH HARDER HARDER HARDER.*"

116

I'm blowing an earth ball into being, breathing life into Adam, blowing a huge tunnel of air into being, holding it steady for you to pass through. I am the North Wind of children's fairy tales; cheeks apuff. Strange. I'm shitting you out, very slowly, as I maintain you in the steady air tunnel that is my body. *Drama is in the endurance, not in the sudden sprint. Not in the high note. Blind stamina is mother to our species.*

Shifra: "STOP. STOP. WAIT. JUST HOLD IT. Get Frédéric back here right now."

"THE BABY'S COMING! THIS BABY'S COMING OUT!"

David: From now on, it looked like a movie. Everyone put on paper outfits and shoe covers. PUSH. NOW, he told you. Suddenly I saw this sticky hair which I knew wasn't yours because it was a different color.

I've flown away, flapping my wings, on the ceiling. I can't see what's happening. It's over for me.

"HERE'S THE BABY!"

"THE BABY'S HERE!"

Baby: "Ahhhhhhhhhhhhhhhhhhhhhhhhhhhhhh . . . "

It's you! It's you! The baby in my October dream. This is unbelievable. You *are* blond! You want a name that begins with *A* . . . Oh! You're so naked! I've never seen anyone this naked. Mother-naked . . .

Give him to me! Give me the baby! I want the baby.

David: The cord was wrapped around his neck. They told you to stop pushing. He screamed just as Frédéric cut the cord—and choked on his own mucus. They couldn't open the first tank of oxygen. The nurses rushed him into the next delivery room. Frédéric left right after you delivered the placenta.

Where's the baby? Why can't I have him?

David. "They're cleaning him up. You'll have him in a minute. Don't worry."

What's that? Let me see it. Let me have it. I'm fascinated by the placenta. Large, liver-like. I want to eat it, keep it. I call for it again and again. The nurse brings it to me. Do I think it's you?

Where's the baby? Is there a baby?

What is this new and terrible pain? A raw burn. Shifra is sewing my anus shut. Stitch by stitch.

Why does it feel like she's cutting me with a razor? My episiotomy? When, why did I get one? Where's the baby? There is a baby, isn't there? Have I given birth or not?

Ah, Here you are. You are. Here.

BABY: DON'T LOOK SO WORRIED. EVERYTHING'S FINE. YOU'RE BACK HOME. WE CONNECTED: TWO TRAPEZE ARTISTS WITHOUT A NET . . .

Oh, baby. Washed up on shore so naked. Come, flop onto my warm belly-beach. Come, creep into the crook of my arm-tree. Climb higher. Nuzzle me. There's wet fruit to eat. Don't stop. Come closer. Eye to eye, soul to soul. Come say hello to your new-born mother.

Your birth is incredible, a miracle. Specific. Real. There is nothing else like it. Like you.

Shifra: "We have to take him now. . . ."

You're gone. Gone. It's as if you don't exist.

I lie here without you, being sewn up. Alone. So alone. The wall clock reads 6:00 A.M..

One hour later. I float up and down the hospital corridor, ten pounds lighter. Exuberant.

You are a bloody miracle. That which is incomprehensible—but so. You exist. You really exist. But how? I knew I was pregnant, but I never believed that you'd pass through me into being.

Little miracle: Wake up! Wake up!

"Visiting hours are over. He'll have to leave," the nurse says, averting her face from the sight of your father. A Mother Superior avoiding the sight of a naked man.

"David's the father," I explain. "He's rooming in."

"Oh, is he? I'll just have to check that," she says.

"Don't worry, there won't be any sex. Ever again," I call after her.

Evening: We drink champagne, laughing. Quietly. Why isn't there a double bed here? Your father has to sleep on a small army cot.

Little one: What are *you* doing right now? Do you want to come to a party? We could steal you. . . .

"This is a stickup. We want *him*. No-name over there!" (Strange, how hospitals make you feel criminal for having normal emotions.)

Baby: You could have roomed in with us. But the room is so tiny. We could have insisted on leaving tomorrow. But I'm too exhausted to go anywhere.

The truth is I chose this time to rest. Apart from the world. Apart from you.

I'm terrified of being alone with you.

Still. Our separation is unnatural. What we need is a very large room—two rooms really—with an experienced mother living in. I want to be able to run in and make sure you exist. Once every hour.

January 7, 1978

9:00 A.M.: "He's here," I tell my mother. "Come." I've waited a full day before calling her.

"I know," she says. "I was just leaving now. I'll be there soon."

Here, Mother. Here is your grandchild. Made by me. Who was made by you. Will you love me now? Will you love him more? Will you live with us and be my love?

"He doesn't look like anyone we know," she says, looking at you through two glass barriers.

"He looks like himself," I say.

I want to hand you to her. I want to see her hold you. (I want to imagine it's me she's holding.)

But babies aren't allowed in the rooms during visiting hours. Even for grandmothers.

Tomorrow: no visitors, no phone calls. Tomorrow I have to name you.

Will I ever sit again? My anus is shut in horror. My vagina no longer exists. I'm sore.

I'm afraid to look at my stitches. I look. They're a jagged line, veering off, grinning madly down, below my vagina.

Throw away the textbooks! I think I've discovered the secret of maternal personality. After you give birth, you never shit again. You don't dare to. And you never tell anyone why you keep smiling so mysteriously.

Today I'm spending the afternoon locked in the bathroom. Alone. To decide on your name. To summon up the courage to shit.

You don't look like a Daniel (your pre-chosen name). There's something fierce and tawny about you. You're the Lion! You're *Ariel:* God's Lion. You'll be my father Leon's namesake—and for *your* father, you'll have a Hebrew name.

I dub thee Ariel, faery spirit of my tempest. You'll be my Jerusalem. . . .

I'll name you David too. It won't be mispronounced as often.

Ariel David. Arr-i-*elle* Da-*veed*.

Ah! What pleasure! The beauty of your name.

The fact that I can shit again.

Too much to do. We watch a video cassette movie about taking care of babies. I take notes. A nurse comes to teach us how to bathe and clean you. A hundred people have to be called. A rabbi has to be found for the *bris* (religious circumcision). People invited. I have to arrange a Women's Ceremony for you. All in the next four days.

I have to breast-feed you. Every four hours. With what? I have thin gruel, right out of *Oliver Twist.* The nurses must be feeding you. You don't suck that hard.

I hold you awkwardly. A huge-breasted failure.

January 9, 1978

The nurses make your father put on a surgical mask and gown when they bring you in. I wander around disheveled. Dark circles under my eyes. But I'm the mother. I don't need a mask.

I lay you across my stomach. You could still fit inside me. But you're outside.

My body thinks it's still pregnant with you. I may not be willing to give birth to you for . . . how long?

Tomorrow we leave. What do babies wear in a snowstorm?

January 10, 1978

My little bride, my only bride, I carry you across the threshold. You're dressed in white: lace crochet and satin trim. I hand you over to your father, who hands you over to Frances, your baby nurse. Bless Frances for being here! (Why do you need a nurse? Are you sick?)

Frances coos over you. She undresses and redresses you. She brings you in to me for breast milk.

What? I'm sitting on the edge of the bed, holding a shoe in one hand. Thinking.

How can I be so frightened of you? You're so tiny! I'm more frightened of you than of anyone else I know. If you knew this, you'd laugh, or really cry.

Ariel: Welcome to your second home on Earth.

January 12, 1978

I dream of your sudden death. The stopped breath. The violent choking. The mysterious convulsion. My fear paralyzes me. I don't want to come near you when I'm poisoned by such imaginings.

Only you can comfort me. By remaining alive. I dread your cries. I crave them.

You fall on my breast, fiercely, like a lion. When you lose my nipple, you rage, grow desperate. Sightless, you burrow for it in my shoulder, under my breast. Frantic, ridiculous.

This is a matter of life and death for you. You clarify human nature for me.

Such peace, when I breast-feed you. Such pleasure! When you put a hand to my nipple, I tingle, I flush. There is no end, no rude climax to this sensation. You suck on my nipple and I feel it in my clitoris and all along my soul.

When will you and I be satisfied like this again?

Will this nightmare ever end?

Your repertoire of hand gestures are—embarrassingly—all mine! You preach Mountain Sermons. You pontificate. Your whole little hand makes Talmudic spirals in the air.

Your testicles fall to your knees. A grandmother's dugs. How can they be so big? You *do* have erections. I watched. You got me in the eye.

You're a toothless grandfather. You're not a baby yet. How long does it take to become one? As long as it takes to become a mother?

Every hour you're being born again. You breathe furiously. Your skin gets blotchier. Your fingers scratch your face, gasping for air.

Asleep, you're an arabesque in pink—oh, so pink—and gold. You look like an angel in a painting. It's clear. The masters used babes at sleep as models for their cupids and other heavenly beings.

Asleep, you seem to be living other lives, remembering terror, power. *Just now, you laughed out loud.* Eerie. Wonderful.

Who are you? How many are you? There is too much to catch hold of. Too many expressions, memories. Yours— and mine too.

January 13, 1978

Dawn. Friday. You have the hands of a violinist. They play over your mouth, worriedly, practicing. Ancient One: Today is your *bris.* Am I doing the right thing? My innocent Isaac: Why do Jewish men need to do this, before accepting a male child into their protective custody? Proclaim love of God first, family second? A ritual wounding, to ward off a more personal one? Patriarchal tampering with what Woman and Nature have made?

Today, blood will flow from the sweetest and tiniest of penises—yours. And I, your mother, will stand by and do nothing to prevent it. I have agreed to it. Your father's desire to do this is so strong, I dare not deny him. I'd be afraid—for you—if I did. I'd be afraid—for my sake, for *our* sake—to protest my anger so firmly. This quarrel is very old. I am powerless.

Baby: Forgive me. *I'd be guilty too.* I cannot cut you off beforehand from this people. *That* severing is your choice, not mine to make for you. (May you never make such a choice. . . .)

Tender One: I'll fast. To protect you. To protest the necessity for this deed. And for my own reasons.

Today, thirteen women gather in your honor to bless you.

8:30 AM.: We've laid out the honey cakes, the fresh bagels. There's sweet wine and harsh, golden whiskey. There's soft white cheese. A mound of bright green olives. Oranges, chocolates, hot coffee.

Outside, the snow whirls.

9:30 AM.: The women come in, cheeks glowing, eyes filled with love. Miriam has flown in from Chicago. Suzanne has come down from Pennsylvania. Carolyn has come from Maryland. The other women have come with great difficulty: from Brooklyn, Long Island, lower Manhattan. The rabbi is here. Your relatives are here. My mother is here.

The rabbi holds the wine aloft, recites the ritual blessing. The men turn white. Frances is poised to spring at the rabbi. Miriam moves to hold my hand. Your father's fists are clenched. My face is turned away.

It's over! The rabbi makes a speech in English. My mother weeps and smiles. Your uncles hold you.

Time for the Women's Ceremony. We go into my study. We sit in a circle on the floor, on large pillows: godmothers, all.

The women will bless you, each in her own voice, each with her own wish. The room is filled with flowers: roses, anemones. I've laid out candles and matches. Miriam holds you. The men watch. Some stop, voluntarily, at the door. Your father joins us.

Miriam begins. She lights one of the candles.

"Women. Let us each, in turn, light a candle for Ariel. Let us bless him with a wish. Let us each give him something of ourselves—a strand of hair, a nail, growing. I'll paste it down for you in this little Book of Life. To seal the wish."

She takes out a pair of scissors, Scotch tape, a folded-over piece of red oaktag. The women are silent. We all watch the first flame.

"May you never know any more pain than you've known today."

"May you never be as lonely as I've been. May you have strong friendships."

"May your parents have the courage to allow you to be yourself. May they love you for it."

"Good health."

"Long life."

"May you be blessed by women all your life, as you are today."

"I wish you playfulness. And laughter."

"I bless you with musical talent."

"Never turn away from your mother. May you know her

as we do. I bless you—and her—in life long friendship together."

"May you love and be loved by your father. May you
be blessed by his sensitivity and his gentleness."

"I hope you have the courage to be the child of feminists.
The strength to be 'different.' I bless you with trusting your
own instincts."

"I bless you with luck. May you be lucky."

"May you honor women in your life, as we honor you
today."

Ariel: Are you listening? You're so quiet in Miriam's
arms, on Frances's lap. You know, we should be naked, gar-
landed. We should each kiss you on every part, every limb.
We should spend the day reclining, eating. Telling stories.

But it's perfect this way too. Just as it is.

"This is what the women do in Yemen!" Eli, from
Yemen, insists. "Where did you learn it?" He is the first
man to speak.

Now I can break my fast. I ask my mother to bring me
some breakfast.

"What kind of breakfast? I don't live with you. I don't
even know how you like your coffee." Is she yelling?

"Just take one thing off each plate and please bring it
to me," I whisper. I think.

"When are you going to send thank you notes to my
friends for their gifts?" she asks, handing me a mug of coffee.

"Why don't you do it for me? It's more than I can handle.
I can't even thank *my* friends. . . ."

"Oh, but you have to. You're a mother now."

"Why don't you help me? Why are you leaving so soon?
Don't leave me!" Am I screaming? Do I say this?

Friends have cleared the food away. They sit, waiting
to keep me company for a while.

"You're always surrounded by strangers," my mother
says bitterly. "You have no time for me. You don't need
me."

"I hate you! How can you do this to me on this day, of all days!" *Which one of us says this?*

We are each stepmother and stepchild; ugly duckling and unwanted relative.

Dark lovers.

Gone. Everyone. I collapse into bed. I can't rest. I'm consumed by my mother's behavior. I call her at midnight.

"Hello. I never want to see you again. You can visit your grandson whenever you want—only warn me first. I'll make sure to be out." (Please say the magic words: "I love you.")

"I'd rather not see him under those conditions. . . . Does this mean I should give back the crib? That I won't be needing it?" (She's somehow acquired a crib.)

"I can't answer that," I say. We both burst into tears, hang up.

January 14, 1978

The maternity store can't deliver any nursing bras for at least two weeks. My one bra is sweat-soaked. What will I do? Your father's list of errands is so huge I can't add to it. Anything "just" for me is not important enough.

The woman who makes the long flowing dresses won't bring any up here.

"Susan," I tell her, "I just can't get out. I'm too tired. The weather's too cold for me. My publisher is sending a photographer over next weekend. I need something to wear. Bring me any three dresses. One size fits all. I'll buy them sight unseen."

"I'm sorry, Phyllis. It's against my policy to take merchandise out. . . . I want you to be happy with my things. I can't pick them for you."

I have nothing to wear. I have no one who can shop for me. It is beyond me to run out into the snow, the bitter cold, to look for fat ladies' clothes. I didn't realize that my tailored clothes would never, never fit me now.

What will I do? What do other new mothers do?

"You wear your maternity clothes for a while," Nora tells me. "Anything that's not completely destroyed, you clean and put on. Thought you'd never have to look at them again, didn't you?"

I should have bought new maternity clothes in December. Next time . . . *Next time?????*

January 16, 1978

You're always hungry. It's always time to feed you. You suck for an hour every two and a half hours. A woman doing this can do nothing else—unless she's allowed to do whatever else it *is* while she breast-feeds.

My friend Clara is chief of a psychiatric ward. Last year she tried to breast-feed on the job. The other psychiatrists, the patients, couldn't handle it. She was accused of sexual exhibitionism! A doctor as a breast-feeding mother is too threatening.

My friend Sharon tells me she used to cover herself with a blanket when she breast-fed in the living rooms of friends! A breast-feeding Mother will not be tolerated.

Topless, bottomless women, dancing in cages; "jiggling" TV actresses, pornographic magazines. Everywhere the female breast is exposed. *But not in a casual and naturally sacred way.* Breast-feeding is still a dirty, private choice. Not a proud public fact.

"Don't do it, Phyllis. It will ruin your breasts," two friends insist.

Ariel: What will happen to us when we start going out?

January 17, 1978

Never have I known such exhaustion. Never. I'm too tired to get out of bed to go to the bathroom. I'm too tired to ask for soup or tea. I'm too tired to drink it when it's brought.

My body won't obey my will. My body is not-me. I have no body to use to get things done.

Every two and a half hours you're brought in to me. I walk to the rocking chair. You feed for at least an hour. I crawl back into bed.

Someone—you, I think—has turned the sound up too high. I jump at whispers. I'm expected to respond constantly. It's beyond my capacity. My entire system is geared for alarm, for emergency. But I'm paralyzed. I'm too sensitive to be in charge of a baby. I'm unfit for ordinary events. How can I protect you in my weakened state?

I am returned from a distant journey. I need to recover. First my naked nervous system. I need a new myelin sheath. I need pure silence to listen to. Someone should bring me special foods.

I need to return to my senses slowly, properly.

I have all the symptoms of battle fatigue.

What if I had to do the cooking, and I felt like this? What if I had another baby tugging at me, and I felt like this? What if I couldn't afford to pay anyone to help me, and I felt like this? What if I didn't have your father home with me? What if I did and it only meant that I had to cook his dinner too?

Would I be this tired if I were twenty and not thirty-seven? Am I still recovering from the flu? Is it the extra sixty pounds? Is it going without sleep for two nights in labor? Is it being in labor for so long? Is it the back labor?

Am I so tired because I'm breast-feeding you?

I have good excuses. But I don't believe them. I feel

like a malingerer, a failure. After so many years of disciplined energy, a stranger emerges from within: a lazy old woman! A cranky baby! A hopeless invalid!

Ariel: I'm undone.

No one sees how exhausted I am.

I don't know how to show it.

Mysteriously, I pull myself together. I feel an impostor. *I am not myself.* Is this how it will be: me, pulled apart, existing on at least two opposing levels at the same time? With no one comprehending all the levels? The level of my longing to be alone with you. The level of my longing to be just as I was before you. My being leveled into fatigue.

I'll "pass" for normal as usual. At what cost?

Can I actually pull it off?

Doesn't everyone see how different I am? Are they just being polite?

Am I permanently split apart? Me in one room? You in another? No longer One?

No longer are young men sent into the wilderness, to return only after a vision has transformed them. Pregnant women, new mothers are. I begin to understand the silence of mothers. I am growing silent. I begin to understand the nervous, nonstop talking of mothers to deny silence.

Under patriarchy, pregnancy and childbirth are savage "tests" of your ability to survive in the wilderness alone. And to keep quiet about what you've seen. Whether you're *accepted* back depends on your ability, your willingness to live without any confirmation that you've undergone a rite of passage. You, who have undergone an experience of total aloneness in the universe. You, who are totally responsible for another life. *You* must keep silent, pretend to return to life as usual.

Is it too dangerous to treat motherhood as so existentially grand an event—*when most men don't become mothers?*

Should I speak, then, in a small voice about small things? The "cute" little baby clothes, the "darling" little baby?

But to become a mother is to open the gates of your womb to admit life—and death—into the world. It is so significant an act, it is *devalued.* Falsely flattered. Lied about. Lived alone.

A woman alone is a Mother.

Can I bear the turning away from me by my mother and by other people, without questioning my sanity, without deciding to die? Can I "swim" and not "sink" as this great silence buzzes around me, louder and louder? Will other mothers confirm my experience? Or will they claim no wilderness, no vision, no transformation? No terrifying solitude? ("It's not that bad. You get over it. I did it. What are you making a fuss about?")

A Mother is a woman alone.

January 10–17, 1978

I take the messages off the answering machines, return ten business calls, open the mail.

I see you at your moment of birth. I'm shocked by how naked you are. Your right profile: sensitive, stubborn. Over and over again, I watch you being born.

I interview two students who want to study with me for school credit. I begin to answer my mail. I dictate everything I can remember about labor and delivery into a tape cassette.

Whenever I'm lying on my back or half lying down, I'm in the delivery room, pushing down, pushing a baby out. Suspended on the ceiling. I'm still there.

I go downtown to see about teaching some courses in Manhattan.

January 18–23, 1978

A meeting with two European feminists. They have such illusions about Feminists and Feminist power in America!

You "bliss out" at my breast. You gulp desperately, then sleep for a minute, startle yourself awake. Then start all over again. Like me in labor with you.

Another bureaucratic mess to untangle! My university claims *not* to have received my grades in the mail. Is this more harassment, or just the usual inefficiency?

A four-hour session with a photographer. Smile for the camera.

My right arm gets numb when I hold you. My lower back hurts, hurts. My feet ache.

January 24, 1978

Work on sending out birth announcements. Your first visit to the pediatrician. (She's wonderful: warm and funny and human.) You've gained a pound since birth. You're an inch and a half longer.

> *Your father is split into three people, fast-motion. He's always out shopping. He's always in the kitchen, unpacking the items. He's always in the bedroom, asking me what I need. He seems to have his coat on all the time.*

Two students come over with late papers. I've promised to read them on the spot so they can graduate.

> *I can't seem to get through a book. My eyes hurt. My attention wanders. I can't even watch a television program from beginning to end.*

January 28, 1978

I see an internist. Do I have anemia? A malfunctioning thyroid again? I have my eyes checked too. Giving birth has shaken my vision: literally.

> *No one realizes I mean to kill myself. I imagine all the ways* you *can die. Then I cry. For you.*

January 30, 1978

"Alan, hello! Glad you're back!" It's my Chairman calling, just back from a month in Europe. "Oh, I'd like to teach, but it's too late," I tell him. "I gave up. I've taken a child care leave: without pay or medical benefits. But I couldn't live with such uncertainty, such harassment."

He's figured out a "plan": I can teach two courses in Manhattan, and one course in Westchester. This way I could breast-feed on my Manhattan days. . . . If I could have been sure of this in December, even in early January! Now, I can't possibly whirlwind myself into a full-time assistant professor in twenty-four hours.

Maybe I could if I hadn't just given birth.

Maybe I wouldn't be as sad as I am if I could have counted on a regular academic schedule. And salary.

January 31, 1978

I've been indoors for 6 weeks. I have to get out. Into the biting cold we go, to hear a friend sing jazz. I still look pregnant: sweatered, trussed up for warmth. Stepping carefully into huge snow dunes, running over ice: looking for a Saturday night taxi.

Ah! Wine, women, song . . .

"Phyllis," your father says, "I'm just going to call the babysitter, make sure everything's okay."

He doesn't return. I find him sitting in the phone booth.

"There's no answer at the apartment," he says. "I'm calling the building. Hello? Hello? Listen, did you see a woman taking a little blond baby out in a basket?"

We fly home. You're sleeping. So is the babysitter. So deeply, she wouldn't hear you—forget about the telephone. *Will I ever sleep like this again? Will David?*

February 1, 1978

Ariel: I imagine all the ways I can kill you.

I can drown you in the bathtub.
I can smother you with a pillow.
I can bang your head on the floor: once, hard.

Last month I wept when I *heard* about a baby dying. This month I do the killing. I kill—and tremble in horror. Why such images?

I'm enraged. *My* life is gone. There is only "us," with you always first. I haven't slept through the night once since you were born.

Perhaps I exorcise my fear of your death by becoming Death's agent: by playing out its possibility myself first.

I imagine your death against my will. Your vulnerability disorders me. You are too helpless, too tiny. How can you survive?

Part Three

MOTHERHOOD

February 5, 1978

Descent into non-industrial time. The rhythm is constant, timeless. Nothing gets "done." I control nothing. The rhythm compels and exhausts me.

I write a lecture I'm giving later this month. The weather is biting, vicious.

Smooth, slightly sour: this is the smell, the feel of you.

Frances is gone. We need to hire a babysitter-housekeeper to help your father when I'm on the road. Today I interviewed twenty-two applicants: all resentful, incompetent. Understandably. What will I do?

February 7, 1978

What a steady little motion you make at my breast. How warm and busy your hands are. Laid flat across my breast, or clutching my finger.

You are hope, unafraid, as you pounce on my nipple. Eyes closed, you suckle fiercely, swiftly, as if demons were at your heels. Sated, you sigh sweetly, groan softly.

Special moments: listening to Dinah Washington sing Bessie Smith while having you at my breast.

I watch little boys on the street now, climbing onto buses, talking to their mothers. There is an earnestness, a sweet-voicedness to them that I never noticed before.

February 8–14, 1978

I'm interviewed at home by a wonderful woman from *Publisher's Weekly.* I go out for a business meeting at my publisher's.

> *I'm plunged into life in the ordinary. Surely, surely, I'll break beneath this load. I feel a mule, a blind Samson going round and round.*

A steady procession of would-be students, baby-sitters, housekeepers.

> *Ariel: You were born with six pounds of invisible laundry that became material only when we got you home. It's accelerated by two pounds each week. My life is a laundromat. My life is a milk bar. My life is a series of unfinished tasks. How long can I keep pretending otherwise?*

February 16, 1978

Peoria, Illinois: Standing on line in the airport, I long for you. My breasts ache for you—literally. I look at your photo. I sigh. It's as if I'm in love.

Two women are standing in front of me in an airport line, holding babies. I smile. One of the women has a six-week-old baby. I move closer. I stare. I make mother conversation. They turn their backs on me. Oh, Ariel. How I miss you.

I'm jealous that your father can stay with you.

I'm jealous that you're getting all your father's attention. Not me. I'm out alone in the world.

I'm angry at myself for not being competent enough to take you along with me. (Even though your pediatrician said I shouldn't, I blame myself for not doing it anyway.)

The women in Kansas City are wonderful. They keep me up half the night with questions and revelations. One woman is wounding, hostile. She gets up to give my lecture a "failing grade."

"You're not as organized as I thought you were," she says smugly. "And there are several important points I'd expected you to go into more deeply. All I can say is I'm disappointed."

Oh, Lady. It's amazing I'm here at all, pacing the platform, rising to passion. If you only knew how lately from childbed I've risen.

February 17, 1978

A large conference in Chicago. Ten men and one lone woman: me. My breasts really ache now. Is there a baby in the house I can nurse? I'd like to ask but don't.

Ariel: I'm hurrying back, the plane is landing—you're at the airport! (How thoughtful your father is.)

Oh, baby, baby. You command my breast fiercely, as we drive back to the city.

How will I manage these separations? Can I take you along? In and out of taxis, on planes, howling on camera? We'll try it. You'll come with me on my next out-of-state trip.

"Let's eat out. I'm starving. We'll take him with us. He's sleeping. If he wakes up I'll just feed him."

Whereupon the owner of the small neighborhood restaurant refuses to seat us.

"Not with a baby. Baby belongs at home."

"I'm not moving until we eat." There's blood in my voice.

"O.K. But he sits on your lap while you eat, Mama. We have no extra chairs for babies. I'm in the restaurant business for money. This is not a park." He grumbles, leads us to a table.

Whereupon a large, drunken customer starts bellowing, demanding more beer. The owner is servile. He doesn't ask him to leave.

"Honey, don't pay him no mind," the waitress says. "He's just nervous. What a nice baby!"

Whereupon I discover that there is no place to change an infant in a public bathroom. I squat, change you on my lap. The bathroom is small, too cold. Someone bangs, impatient to come in. There are no disposable diapers, no baby talc for sale in this bathroom. Come to think of it, have I *ever* seen a baby-changing station in a movie theater, a nightclub, an office building? Do they provide free Tampax in public places, the way they do toilet paper?

Should I run for the Presidency on a platform of free Pampers and Tampax in all public places? Double-width supermarket aisles for shopping with a baby?

There are two women banging on the bathroom door now. They'll have to wait. Where else can I feed you but in here, shivering?

Are mothers and children supposed to remain indoors, invisible? For how many years? What if I had three children four years apart? Am I supposed to stay at home for twelve years?

No. Mothers and children can visit each other. At home. Where we all belong.

Would I want a crying baby near me in a restaurant—especially now that I've got you at home?

February 19, 1978

I'm doing an all-day workshop on women and religion. *You're* at your uncle's house. I call three times just to hear you gurgle into the phone.

Here I am, baby. All ready for you. "Phyllis, Mom left this for you," my brother says.

"What!" I scream. "Did you let your mother in the second I left?" (We haven't seen her since your *bris.*) My brother, my rival. He gives me two large scrapbooks. My mother's been cleaning out her house. A thick lock of auburn hair: my first haircut. Monthly reports from my pediatrician. School report cards. It's all here.

"She hates me," I tell your father. "She wants no part of me. No reminder of me around."

"Phyllis," he says, "she wants to show you how she's kept everything, how she's treasured you. She probably wants to make up. She doesn't know how."

February 22, 1978

Last night, I took you into my bed to play Peek-a-Boo and Hug. This much pleasure must be illegal!

"Phyllis, you really look happy," your father says. "Who would ever have believed it? It's probably safe to love a baby," he muses. "Safer than loving another adult."

"I don't know," I say. "Is this playing peek-a-boo with a nursing infant 'love'? Will Ariel love me forever because tonight we're under my covers together?"

"Phyllis," he says, "I hadn't suspected such maternality in you."

"Maternality?" I say. "I'm having a wonderful time! Ariel doesn't care what I think, or who I know. He's a very basic sort of person. Being with him is the closest I come to' being' with other people."

Is this what other mothers experience, leading them to scorn lesser activities as superficial, boring? Leading them to press motherhood on all women? Leading them to put up with or deny the low valuation of motherhood?

Would I be able to feel such joy if I were trapped with you full-time, Ariel?

February 23–24, 1978

From now on I have to be available to whoever calls and wants to interview me. It's not enough to just write a book. If you're *lucky,* you have to promote it, without pay, for three to six months before and after a publication date.

> *I begin to menstruate for the first time in twelve months. It's as if nothing has happened. Has my body forgotten you already?*

The phone rings constantly. I'd like to run away, be alone with you. I can't.

> *Sleepless nights. You have gas cramps, constipation. You scream. And scream. Your father walks you. I can't sleep. How will I get through tomorrow?*

February 27, 1978

The child care problem: *it exists.* The child care solution: it doesn't.

In the beginning, before you were born, your father and I decided that he'd be the "mother" and I'd be the "mother's helper." For seven weeks we've *been* your mothers—with help from Frances in January.

Two mothers, both of whom need to do other work—even with paid help—aren't enough for one new baby. Your demands crush both of us.

How can this be?

You need a minimum of six mothers. Where can I find four other reliable Mother surrogates?

Hello, Baby Nurse Employment Agency? Please send over four part-time child care workers. Warm people, with some feminist awareness, please. Two men, two women . . . What? I'd have to pay each one a full-time salary of one hundred and seventy-five dollars? For five days? *No problem.* That's only seven hundred dollars a week. A thousand dollars weekly, if we include weekends. Domestic chores, laundry, shopping, are extra? *No problem.*

I'll just hold up a bank, get arrested, thrown into jail. And all my problems will be solved.

February 28, 1978

When I insist I'm depressed, suicidal, friends look worried—and look away.

What if I don't "make it"? What if I only pretend to pull myself together? What if everyone settles for my pretense?

I grow mistrustful, silent. Why try to share what I feel? It disturbs people too much. It reminds mothers of their own drowning, long repressed.

Ariel: *I may never recover from this amount of responsibility.* How do other mothers, with fewer resources than I, manage? Do they ever recover? Health, hope, private time?

*M*arch 1, 1978

I sleep better when I breast-feed.

Giving you a bath: swimming, you grin loudly, lopsidedly, splashing with all your tiny might.

Ariel: Will you remember any of this?

In his image: Is it possible that men would have all snowflakes look alike? Nature is being lazy when a child looks exactly like his father; when a child looks exactly like her mother. This is the bizarre right of kings: mass-produced coins. Each child should look only like himself.

So I tell myself, Ariel, realizing that you don't look like me or your father. Yet.

March 3, 1978

Ariel: You've taken over the entire apartment. I used to have it: with a desk in every room, file cabinets in all the clothes closets, books in the kitchen.

You outdo me—with your stroller in one corner, a carriage in the entranceway. Each room is decorated in your laundry. It lies in piles, all the way to the overflowing laundry basket. Used diapers fill every wastepaper basket.

There's more: A collapsible playpen. A musical infant swing. Boxes of diapers. Cartons of formula. Blankets, quilts. Your garments.

Your toilette and pharmaceutical items: That tiny comb. Nose drops. Aspirin. Paregoric. Vaseline. Vitamin drops. Eye ointment. Tissues. Desitin. Balmex.

Since I—and an assistant—work in the living room, we pretend these things aren't here.

How did my mother survive with three children in an apartment half the size of ours?

March 4, 1978

Alone together with your father for the first time since you were born. We check in overnight at a Manhattan hotel. I need to practice reentry as a "normal" adult outside the home, away from you.

We can see the skyline from the swimming pool. We "dine" very slowly, to music. There's fur on the bed, chrome everywhere. Muted lights. But "sex" is impossible. I'm shy, like a sexually repressed young girl.

Does Motherhood the Virgin make?

Gone, gone is my Mediterranean lust. "Sex" is beside the point. "Sex" is a habit. The longer I go without it, the longer I *can* go without it. Sex is nothing compared to the miracle of your existence. Sex is dangerous: *it works.*

I don't want to get pregnant. I do too.

Another child would kill me. Now the prospect of an abortion is as traumatic as the prospect of going through a pregnancy unwanted, unmanageable. How painful it must be for *mothers* to have abortions! Forced to by poverty, by wisdom. Who can afford to have ten children? Martyrs—and millionaires?

Tonight your father and I hug—and fall asleep like brother and sister. I feel guilty to be away from you, *in pursuit of my own pleasure.*

*M*arch 7, 1978

"I'll fail everything in school if I don't get some real relief," David yells. "I fell asleep in class yesterday. I can't concentrate at all."

"O.K." I scream. "You want me to stop earning money? How will we survive? You promised you'd take care of the baby, full-time. But you're not. *Not the way women do . . .*"

"You're the real baby," he screams back. "I have to worry about whether you get to the airport on time. I have to worry about what your mother said to you. Who's attacked you in public today . . ."

Ariel: Your father is extraordinary with you. More efficient than I am. He bathes you, burps you, expertly. He wakes the instant you cry. He reads Dr. Spock every night. His diapers always stick. Mine sometimes come undone.

Your father's efficiency with you will win him more respect than mine would ever win me. More respect than I get from having a calling, or for supporting myself and a family. But not enough respect to socially sanctify him as your mother: *the one with the bottom-line responsibility.* Already people whisper to me about the "fragile male ego." People tell me he'll grow depressed, impotent. Would they worry about my depression?

"He'll run away," my neighbor tells me.

Ariel: How can I take care of you and be the sole breadwinner too? I can't. Breast-feeding four times a day is all I can manage. With enormous difficulty. *It takes four full hours.*

"What does your husband do?" a reporter asked me yesterday.

"Right now he's taking care of our son," I tell her.

"Oh, really?" she said, her face coming undone. Disbelief. Disapproval.

"Phyllis," my brother says on the phone. "How can you trust your baby to someone else?"

"Who are you talking about?" I ask.

"David may mean well, but he's not a woman."

March 8, 1978

Ariel: Happy International Women's Day to you and yours. I lecture in Kentucky tonight.

Suddenly, airborne, I accept the fact of my out-of-body experience during labor. "I" hovered right over my head, connected in an arc to my belly button. My memory of that hovering remains vivid. I can return there at will, as if it's still going on. This would explain why I don't remember certain things your father said happened during labor. *I wasn't there. They didn't happen to me.*

The literature on astral projection notes that it occurs spontaneously when relaxation is enormous, or when the body is overwhelmingly preoccupied with something else— usually with pain. When it occurs spontaneously, it's experienced as "traveling" from the head.

I wonder how many women in labor have experienced this without naming it? (I resisted admitting it to myself for two months.) I wonder how drugs during labor interfere with this phenomenon?

March 10, 1978

My exhaustion, my depression, linger on. I'm afraid I'll collapse.

I go to see a nutritionist, who's more interested in *your* health, baby, than in mine.

"You give him formula-milk?" he yells at me. "Your son's entire mental and physical health is at stake. You're making him a sugar addict. He'll get all the childhood allergies. He'll grow up neurotic like everyone else."

High above me, where I stand accused, the nutritionist smiles. "I know you don't want this to happen. Tell me the reason you can't breast-feed all the time. . . .Oh, you have to travel a lot? O.K. No problem. Get a goat. Goat's milk is next best to yours."

"Goat's milk?" I laugh. "Where would the goat live? In the bathtub? It's filled with laundry."

"O.K. Forget the goat." He makes a reluctant concession. "Go and get a prescription for unpasteurized goat's milk from your pediatrician. If you can. They're all part of the sugar conspiracy."

Ariel: Should I cancel everything and study nutrition? I don't disagree with what this man says. Taking our health seriously takes so much time and money, so much real self-love, it's almost un-American. (Please don't smoke. No meat, please, I'm a vegetarian. No, I don't drink alcohol. I don't eat cake. No fast-food for me, thanks.)

March 11, 1978

A publicity schedule is a politician's schedule. (Actually, it's a mother's schedule too.) You repeat yourself over and over again. Every day. At top speed. Whatever you happen to want or feel is irrelevant. And you're not supposed to complain. Somewhere, there are women dying to be in your maternal shoes. Somewhere, there are authors who aren't even *published,* much less publicized. Smile! You're on.

Ariel: Shall I appear on television as a disheveled mother? If I sit there on camera with a vacant, depressed stare, will mothers everywhere see themselves, and rejoice in confirmation? Or will the studio guard refuse to admit me? Will they say of me that I've become . . . a mother? Will they take away my books, my doctorate? Will they give me a cotton housedress and tell me not to bother them for twenty years?

I feel the impostor when I sweep into the public world now. No longer all of a piece. Wherever I am, a "piece" (is it you?) is missing, invisible.

I know that somewhere there must be mothers who in one week go back to their regular clothes; who appear at their desks as if nothing ever happened, whistling.

*M*arch 13, 1978

Together, in the Midwest, on TV. *I can't handle it.* You, your feedings—and doing publicity. The Fuller Brush Feminist with fallen arches is back again: smiling.

On the road, there's never enough sleep. Never any privacy. No time for a walk or a shit or a talk with a friend. *No time to breast-feed.*

"Help, America!" I want to say. Just because I'm larger than your own lives on prime-time television today, saying such smart and sassy things, doesn't mean I can handle motherhood. *That's a very good question, I say instead. I'm glad you asked me that.*

America! Women! Do you think I'm not drowning in this transformation into motherhood? *Instead, I point out that the biggest complaint women have about men is not that men are physically violent, but that they're emotionally passive, distant.*

Women! Parents! We're alone in this task. Who mothers mothers? Who mothers parents? I want to ask. *It's crucial for men to be seriously involved in childcare, I say instead, for their sake, as well as for the sake of women and children.*

Ariel: Never have I missed a plane in my life. I did last night, running with you in a basket, down the airport corridor, losing diapers all the way. I couldn't sleep all night. I'm not sure I made sense on TV today.

I can't take you with me again. I'd need a nurse—or your father—to watch you while I worked and while I slept. I haven't the money for two airplane tickets to see America.

Bye, Baby. Bye, bye.

March 16, 1978

7:30 A.M. Television taping
2:00 P.M. First newspaper interview. At home
4:30 P.M. Second newspaper interview. At home
8:30 P.M. Book and author lecture at political club

Nothing seems to work. For example: any part-time baby-sitter hired to look after you automatically comes to me with all her questions. "Do you think his eye looks better?" "Should I put this nightgown on, or do you prefer a stretch suit?" Long after your father has explained that I'm working at home and shouldn't be disturbed—ever—still, she comes to my desk, holding you. Automatically, I reach for you, my concentration broken. Perched on my desk, the woman makes "small talk"—talk she's not used to making with a man.

When I lock the door, the woman feels puzzled, rejected. I can feel her judgment.

Why don't I just give it all up? The interviews, the lectures, the serious writing. Disconnect the phone, unbecome myself? Maybe I'd go crazy, but at least I'd have *one* job driving me nuts, not ten.

March 20, 1978

10:00 A.M. Radio Show
12:30 P.M. TV Show
 5:30 P.M. TV Show. Out of town.

My agent, Samantha, takes me out for a quiet dinner, to celebrate the publication of my book, the child of my soul: the "other" child I grew and wrestled with, long before you were conceived.

The process is totally different.

A book is not an infant. An infant is not a book. Only a mother who writes would know this—or think of comparing the two.

Last year this would never have occurred to me.

March 25, 1978

It has begun. Quietly and without dramatics. My mother and I are speaking again. Somehow she's agreed to take you overnight this weekend. (Did I ask her to? Did she offer it? I can't say.)

I'm so desperate for a breathing space at home, *alone* for a night, that I'm grateful to her.

She's having an experienced grandmother sleep over with her. *She's terrified.* She asks me the same questions over and over again. (What to do if you choke. What to do if you have diarrhea. What to do if you won't eat.)

"Hey, Ma. Relax," I say. "You have three living children. Proof of your superb maternal efficiency."

"I'm an old woman. I don't know if I can handle it. What will you do if I hurt him?"

"You won't hurt him." The question shocks me.

"How terrible your parents are," she croons to you as we leave. "How can they leave you? How can your mother bear to part with you?"

Does she hear what she's saying? Probably not.

*M*arch 27, 1978

Whether I'm describing the chores of child care or of book care, this is what I'm told:

"Phyllis, it can't be all that bad. After all, look how many others have done it and never said a word." Female "macho": stiff upper lip all the way to the loony bin.

Of course women are silent. The job of being a "good" woman, a "tough" broad, involves hiding how much work or pain goes into doing it.

Mothers are allowed to share the details of child care by being "funny."

"You see, there I was holding on to one kid with one hand, the shopping in my other hand, the dog leash with my foot, and with my third arm grabbing for the kid that got away."

But when this is happening, the terror of losing the baby, the groceries, the dog isn't funny.

*A*pril 1, 1978

April, this "cruelest month" . . . Ariel, I'm home for only five days. Your father and Natalie (newly arrived) are caring for you.

Los Angeles, San Francisco, Chicago, Boston, Baltimore, Philadelphia—and New York television studios—will claim me for twenty-three days straight. Two days lecturing in Connecticut and California will help pay our bills.

I flew out to Los Angeles yesterday. *I wish you were here.* Will it matter if I'm not with you for a while now? You're so little. What can you possibly remember?

We'll have a fat green summer together. I promise!

Don't believe me, Ariel. I'll always have something else to do.

*A*pril 2, 1978

I'm sitting on the balcony of my Los Angeles hotel room, trying to forget you're not here. My breasts ache.

I'm being interviewed by two magazine writers. I smile. I gesture expansively. I repeat myself.

Ariel: I feel a failure for not bringing you along. I'm superwoman—right? I should be able to breast-feed you, go without sleep, and do a fifteen-hour media day with no trouble. Trouble is, I can't. Trouble is, I'm guilty because I feel my "place" is as much here, helping the book, as it is at home with you.

Weaning time. For both of us.

Monday, April 3, 1978

Wake-up call	7:00 A.M.	
Pickup at hotel	8:00 A.M.	
Arrive	8:45 A.M.	TV Show (live)
		On: 9:00 A.M.
		Out: 10:00 A.M.
Pickup	10:15 A.M.	
Arrive	11:15 A.M.	Radio Show (live)
		On: 12:00 P.M.
		Out: 1:00 P.M.
Pickup	1:00 P.M.	
Arrive	1:15 P.M.	TV Show (live)
		On: 2:00 P.M.
		Out: 2:45 P.M.
Pickup	2:45 P.M.	
Arrive	3:30 P.M.	Newspaper Interview
		(restaurant)
		On: 3:30 P.M.
		Out: 4:30 P.M.
Pickup	4:30 P.M.	
Arrive	5:30 P.M.	Newspaper Interview
		(hotel room)
		On: 5:45 P.M.
		Out: 7:00 P.M.

"Hello, hello! How's Ariel? What did he eat today? *All* the egg custard? And his bowel movement? Did he go for a walk?"

Do you know I'm gone? Do you miss me? Do you wonder what happened to your, my, our breast?

I drink too much tonight.

Tuesday, April 4, 1978

Wake-up call	8:30 A.M.	
Pickup at hotel	9:30 A.M.	
Arrive	10:00 A.M.	TV Show (live)
		On: 10:30 A.M.
		Out: 11:00 A.M.
Arrive	11:15 A.M.	Radio Show (tape)
		On: 11:35 A.M.
		Out: 12:30 P.M.
Arrive	12:45 P.M.	Newspaper Interview
		(lunch)
		Out: 1:15 P.M.
Arrive	1:45 P.M.	Radio Show (live)
		On: 2:00 P.M.
		Out: 2:30 P.M.
Arrive	4:00 P.M.	Pre-interview with
		Network TV
		Out: 4:30 P.M.
Arrive	5:00 P.M.	Pre-interview with
		Network TV
		Out: 5:30 P.M.
Arrive	7:00 P.M.	Magazine Interview
		(Part I)
		On: 7:15 P.M.
		Out: 9:00 P.M.

Spinning. It's all spinning around. What am I doing here?

"Hello? It's me. Sorry I'm so late. I literally didn't have a minute. Tomorrow I can't be reached. I'm giving a lecture and workshop, somewhere between here and San Francisco. I'll call you. Not late. I promise. Bye, bye."

Thursday, *April 6, 1978*

Wake up	8:00 A.M.	
Pickup	9:00 A.M.	
Plane	10:00 A.M.	
Arrive		
San Francisco	11:00 A.M.	
Arrive	11:45 A.M.	TV Show (live)
		On: 12:00 P.M.
		Out: 12:30 P.M.
Arrive	1:00 P.M.	Radio Show (live)
		On: 1:05 P.M.
		Out: 1:30 P.M.
Arrive	2:00 P.M.	Radio Show (tape)
		Out: 2:15 P.M.
Arrive	2:30 P.M.	Two Phone Interviews
		(hotel)
		Out: 3:15 P.M.
Arrive	3:30 P.M.	Radio Interview
		(tape: hotel)
		Out: 5:30 P.M.
Arrive	6:50 P.M.	Radio Show (live)
		On: 7:00 P.M.
		Out: 8:00 P.M.
Arrive	9:00 P.M.	Dinner with friend
		(live)
		On: 9:00 P.M.
		Off: 11:00 P.M.

"Hello, hello! Yes, I know it's midnight. First minute . . . I have to fly back to Los Angeles tomorrow for an afternoon newspaper interview. Publicity thinks it's important. I'm coming home Saturday night. First plane I can get."

I don't sleep all night. How will I get through tomorrow?

*A*pril 9, 1978

Back home. Ariel. I've been away for ten days. I haven't thought about you for hours at a time. Is this why you won't take my breast?

Ariel: Did farmers, queens, servants, priestesses, factory workers, prostitutes, merchants, slaves, all personally attend to their own babies twenty-four hours a day?

Ariel: Look at me. It's only two hundred and forty hours. I can still squeeze milk out of my breasts. . . .

Ariel: Was the last time the last time for us then?

*A*pril 15, 1978

"I stayed home for the first year," Judy tells me. "I got crazy. Being with a baby *all the time* is too limiting for any adult. The boredom coupled with the crushing responsibility kills you."

"I feel like that after only a day with Ariel. I'd be a basket case after a week. How did you get around?" I ask her.

"Fine," she answers. "No problem there."

"You mean there were places to change her when you shopped? Child care centers wherever you visited?"

Judy's face grows still.

"I remember one rainy afternoon, long after lunch," she says, "when the museum wouldn't let me in. A baby stroller is a fire hazard, they said.

"They asked me to leave the public library. *The place was empty except for me.* The baby was fast asleep. But the stroller's a fire hazard. . . . *The butcher wouldn't let me in.* Leave the carriage outside. Don't block my doorway, he said. I felt filthy."

I see the remembered humiliation, the anger, on her face.

*A*pril 30, 1978

My mother screeches with delight when she sees you. Those kisses, those exclamations, as I stand by and watch, ever the stepchild.

What do women want? Our mothers.

Clearly, you're my gift to her. (Is that who you are?)

I watch her with you, thinking: This is the woman who taught me to read. This is the woman who *never went out* except to funerals and weddings for nearly fifteen years. She might have been a ballet dancer, but her family wouldn't let her study "such nonsense." She might have been a schoolteacher, but they wouldn't let her go to college. "Nonsense" again, when her earnings and nursing abilities were needed at home. There were sick parents to care for, nieces and nephews to baby-sit for.

"What's wrong with this? Did I do anything wrong by helping my mother?" she asks me. "You should learn from my example," she concludes.

Never is she consciously angry about a life of maternal self-sacrifice. She is only "angry" with me because I'm not like her.

Oh, Mother: What if I can never forgive you?

A friend, visiting, tells me that my mother's eyes follow me all around the room, look away only when I look at her.

I don't believe this.

May 1, 1978

Natalie watches television twelve hours a day. Even while she feeds you. And while she does her needlepoint. A peevish, tiny woman.

Natalie feeds you lovingly. Sings to you. She sits alone on the park bench. Staring straight ahead. Clutching a plastic purse with one hand, the carriage bar with the other. Like a plaster sculpture.

Natalie is "reliable." For the last month she's returned every weekday morning. This has kept me silent, appreciative. Your father fights with her over the consistency of your egg custard, the amount of Desitin she does or doesn't apply. I keep more distance. But I try to talk to her about the television.

"I don't do housework," she tells me. "I can't shop. That and watch a baby too! I can't leave his carriage outside the supermarket. What if he falls out? What if someone steals him? I won't struggle inside with it."

"No, no, Natalie, I'm talking about watching television all day, all night. It's bad for the baby, it's bad for you. I can't stand the noise."

"Well, what should I do all those hours he's sleeping? Tell me that!"

"Straighten up the kitchen?" I ask.

"I won't do it!"

May 5, 1978

Housework, cooking, shopping—child sentry-duty—each dwarf me, shame me. I can't find a solution, personal or otherwise, to the "problem" of domestic maintenance and child care. Who can?

Why is everyone so quiet about this? Why don't the headlines scream "Child Care Emergency" daily? Why are the single-income families silent about the systematic "drowning" of mothers into housewifery and child care? The "drowning" of fathers into money-earning? Why are the two-career, two-income families silent about the emotional sterility of hard-drive careers—as if there's been no miracle, no child? Silent about the high cost and uneven quality of paid mother-surrogates?

Silent—for the same reasons I am. *I'm afraid of being called selfish (for complaining), stupid (for wanting to stay home—or for having to leave home to earn money), really stupid (for having expected to be spared this problem), incompetent (for not being able to solve this dilemma), a "trivializer" (of the romance of motherhood), a "whiner" (about what every other mother takes for granted, knew about all along, handles magnificently. Without complaint).*

I'm afraid of attracting the bitter envy of those less fortunate than me. As hard as I'm finding this passage into motherhood, at least your health is good; at least I can and do earn money, however insecurely; at least! your father is involved in caring for you.

So what if my caring for you *or* my working to pay for baby-sitters makes it impossible for me to write? Where is it written that I must write? How many women, mothers, parents write? Has anyone died of not being-able-to-write? *I would.*

Ariel, my book tour's nearly over. From now on, you're stuck with us. No more hit-and-run baby-sitters, housekeepers, nurses. Somehow—how?—David and I will take care of you and of the house: in shifts, side by side, together.

*M*ay 15, 1978

Shopping lists, laundry loads, piles everywhere, nothing finished. How can I enjoy your sweet babble, when it takes eight full hours a day to "service" you, sixteen to "guard" you? Bottle feeding, diaper changing, vitamins, playing; diaper changing, solid food, dressing; a walk outside, diaper changing. Playing. Food. A bath. More feeding. Getting you to nap, getting you to sleep. Your laundry.

I made a mistake. I'm dying, slowly. My body isn't the same. My lower back always hurts. My throat aches so badly I can't speak. I always have a bad cold. Each night: panic. Each morning: sadness.

I'm irritable, exhausted.

Without energy. So much responsibility: a dull weight flattening me. My soul is gray, apathetic. I make no dramatic threats. I go through my days stunned, bitter, like an animal trapped into laborious captivity, like a prisoner of war.

I can't feel like this and write–lecture–see patients–attend meetings. I doubt I could take care of you full-time, for eight hours and do anything else but recover.

Who can? I could visit you the way traditional fathers and mothers do, for one cautious hour each evening. I don't think that would hurt you. But it would rob me—of what? Your love? Social approval? This chance to be a "real mother"?

Maybe my standards for work are too high. Maybe with your coming I've got to lower them. I can't.

It's only been ten days since I'm really sharing you full-time with your father.

May 17, 1978

Caring for you full-time feels like I've been tackled by a two-hundred-pound weight—permanently. I'll never get used to it. This utter loss of mobility, this heavy responsibility. How can a fifteen-pound human being weigh two hundred pounds?

"It's too hard. I can't go on," I tell my friend Miriam. "It's Ariel—plus having to worry about money, about space, about never being alone . . ."

"I had a one-year-old when I gave birth for the second time," she says.

"Twins? Impossible," I say. "How did you do it?" I ask her.

"It's very hard," she whispers. "You don't sleep. You become peculiar. The grandmothers don't stay. They go back home. 'Don't leave me,' I begged my mother—but she did. You wear old clothes. You make mistakes."

"But where was their father?"

"Oh, he's a wonderful man. He worked fourteen hours a day to support us. Every night, he came home exhausted, late. . . . I knew no one in the city. I lived alone among strangers, the children and I."

"That's why you moved back to Chicago," I whisper.

"It was impossible among strangers," Miriam says simply, the pain darkening her eyes.

May 20, 1978

My sex life is over. I have no energy to masturbate. Whenever I quiet my night insomnia or boredom with a vibrator, my orgasm is without pleasure.

Am I so afraid of getting pregnant again?

Am I disinterested in orgasms that don't lead to pregnancy?

Did my episiotomy flatten my sexual affect? Did giving birth shock my body into silence?

Am I just too tired? Am I too angry—about everything—to allow myself this tiny release?

Sex isn't a good enough release. I need time. Solitude. My own room. Economic security.

Where, now, is my Mediterranean lust? Will it return only if I become pregnant again?

How many other new mothers have no sexual desire? Is it only me?

May 21, 1978

My friend Suzanne, newly pregnant, turns to me as an expert on becoming a mother.

"Phyllis," she says, "I'm angry with Rob all the time. What if I stop painting?"

"You're beginning to feel you don't control your life anymore." I respond. "You're afraid of becoming vulnerable, becoming even more dependent on Rob. What if he fails you?"

She grows quiet, listens.

"Suzanne, when I was pregnant I was terrified for similar reasons. *You just didn't notice.* But look: I'm meeting deadlines. David hasn't failed me. We fight: a lot. I'm not *happy. . . .*"

"What if I love the baby more than I love Rob?" Suzanne asks. "What if he loves the baby more than he loves me? Do you love Ariel more than you love David?" she challenges me.

"No. Not yet."

"Are you sorry you did it?" she asks. Intelligently. Urgently.

"Yes," I answer. "I'm trapped. I can't take Ariel back, or move away from him."

A long silence.

"No," I say. "I'm blessed now."

The infuriatingly ambivalent answers of mothers about mother-hood. No wonder women don't "hear" what mothers say until after-ward, when they hear themselves speaking as mothers.

May 22, 1978

My baby has palms of satin, satin-palms has he.

Ariel: I no longer make lists of where to live and what your needs will be for ten years: play groups, athletics, music lessons, casual contact with nature, religious education, etc. etc.

I'm learning to take one day at a time. I'm beginning to trust life to go on without my having to control it. As if I could! Just as "I" wasn't needed during labor, when a force deeper, more ancient than my own will took over. You are more resilient, less determined by human will than I suspected. You live. You flourish. You do not die.

I am Atlas, holding up an entire world: you. Something holds me up too.

May 24, 1978

Last night you woke up, screaming. Was it a nightmare? Are you re-living a previous death? The sound was eerie, gripping. An innocent infant crying out as though damned.

I believe now in reincarnation.

I believe our "characters" are born with us. I saw your soul at your moment of birth. How can I deny this?

As I stand over your crib, you wake up suddenly and see me there. Is this where we get our idea that a God exists above us, watching over us?

Why isn't God remembered as a woman, then?

May 30, 1978

Two small children are spending the weekend with us. How it changes you! You gurgle and smile valiantly. You make yourself known in every way you can. "Here I am!" you scream, delighted. "Play with me. I exist!"

Ariel: You should be surrounded *every day* by Short People. How can I arrange this? Where is a nearby courtyard filled with sun and small children? Where a common well, a dining hall?

Betty, the children's mother, functions at the center of disorder and steady demand. There is something seductive, something disgusting about it. It reminds me too much of my own childhood: of mothers and children glued together.

"Hey, let me take Ariel out with me for a walk," Betty insists. "He's really a friendly kid."

Your father motions me to one side. "I like Betty. Where did you say you met her? Can we trust Ariel with her? What if she's having a good time with her own kids and forgets about Ariel? She's pretty easygoing."

"I think she's a real mother-person," I say. "You don't trust Ariel out of your sight, do you?"

"Hey you guys! Can I take him out or not?" Betty asks, hugging David.

"Sure," your father says. "Why don't we all go out together? Phyllis, take a break. It's the middle of the afternoon already."

June 3, 1978

Last night Joan asked me if I felt like a mother yet.

"I don't know," I said. "What's a mother supposed to feel like?"

Am I feeling "like a mother" because my life feels inside out—literally? Or because I'm growing quietly obsessed with the importance of seasons, family life, community? Can a stranger TELL I'm a mother by looking at me—when I'm not around?

A mother is *my* mother: not me.

I don't believe you came from my body. The stork brought you. You came in a basket. I found you under a cabbage leaf.

Did you really begin as a single cell? Here you are, outside me; eased loose, set adrift, with no sign of our dark flesh contact.

June 6, 1978

Tonight I visited Emma and her fifteen-day-old son. My arms reached out for that baby, as if I've been holding babies all my life. Strange, that curve of my arm to a new reality, that sympathetic ache in my breasts, when there's a baby in the room. Without words, Emma handed him to me: her miracle.

The erotic smells of a baby: the small, curling-into-you shape of a baby.

Having a child does make you think about your own death. I realize that I don't have a will. Also, who will take care of you, Ariel, if I die? Who will raise you? Whom can I trust?

These are mother-thoughts, but David has them too.

*J*une 8, 1978

Bertha asks me what to do about her teen-age son.

"He's pushing me away—very hard. I try to give him space. Do you think it's a phase?"

This losing of the sons to "manhood." Will you do this, Ariel? Does it matter?

"I don't think of it as a phase," I say. "I see it as a form of psychological matricide."

"He says vicious things to me. 'I hate you.' 'Don't touch me.' He must be suffering terribly."

"So are you. Do you think he'll really kill you off?"

"Oh, no. Not physically! Maybe it's because I'm divorced: Who else can he be angry at? He thinks I prefer his brother. I don't. How can I love one more than the other?"

Guilt. Denial of guilt. Grim truths. Ariel: Will you be an only child? My only child?

June 10, 1978

I sit and watch you playing on the rug, sweet-singer, talking to yourself, rolling over. Know: that at every conception, every birth, there is the most profound ambivalence. (If you ever ask me about this, how will I answer you? Will I turn my face away, soften my answer, minimize the fact that I could have killed you before you were born? That I thought about it, in terrible fascination, often?)

Oh, Ariel! You turn and smile at me just as I write this, comforting me, forgiving me my human nature. Why is so natural a fact: ambivalence, so terrifying that we invent images of perfect maternal love—images that no woman can ever live up to, that no one is ever fooled by? Haunting images.

Suddenly, every woman over thirty who meets me confides in me her desire and her ambivalence about having a child. They say: "I'm afraid it will change the relationship I have with my husband. Does it?"

They say: "I don't want to get married and I don't want to use a man only for his sperm. I haven't much time left. What do you think I should do?"

They ask: "Is it really worth it? Doesn't it tie you down? Haven't you lost your freedom?"

June 11, 1978

"Have another child," my mother says. "You only have a little time left."

How cruel that she should urge me to it again, when she is unable to help me. Does she wish my creative death? Does she hate me for having dared to keep myself for myself so long? Does she really feel that my work is not as important as a child?

I can't just "go out" anymore. I have to plan everything. I must always replace myself before I can be alone—to write, to take a walk. Always, now, I am doubled. (There is me and my surrogate.) Always I am halved. (I am a "pretender" in the world when I go out without you: behaving as I did before—hiding the fact of your existence merely by not mentioning it.)

Ariel: Wherever I am, you're there too, hovering around my shoulders. I'm never alone. Not even when I'm lonely *and* quite alone; in my study, or in another city.

This invasion of my psychic privacy is more jolting than your physical invasion of my time-and-space privacy.

It can only grow as you do. I'm defenseless against you, sweet innocent babe.

June 14, 1978

Suzanne and I have lunch together.

"Phyllis. I'm worried. My best friend, a sculptor, just told me *he* couldn't work for two years after his child was born. He told me to 'wait and see' how I paint after I become a mother. I feel like having an abortion."

I sit up straight. " 'OK, superwoman bitch! Now you'll be brought to your ungrateful and ordinary knees by Nature Herself.' That's what he's saying."

"Exactly. Will I?" she asks me.

"Yes. You will. I have a sense of my human limitations that I totally lacked before," I tell her. "My lower back hurts almost constantly. I'm seeing an acupuncturist for pain control."

"Stop!" she says.

"No. I'm trying to answer you. I couldn't have functioned these last five months if David weren't totally committed to me and Ariel, and if we couldn't afford some household help. *I nearly didn't make it as it is.* The responsibility is awesome, the details overwhelming, and I'm lucky, privileged, compared to most mothers. Be prepared to have your life turned upside down: in unpredictable ways. Probably forever."

"Stop!" she says.

I continue.

"Ariel is a great teacher. Not only does he force me to *see* my limitations; he has me—kicking and screaming—accepting them. *More:* For the first time in my life, I'm learning about love . . . about what it takes to nourish, maintain human life. Giving birth changes how you see the world. You know, when I walk down the street I see each person being born. I exist *in relation* to human vulnerability and nakedness as never before.

"Suzanne, I'll tell you this: It's crucial for a woman, *any* woman, to have her own money and a totally involved father—or "other" person. Without that, I don't see how mothers manage, psychologically or practically."

"Money's not a problem right now," she says. "But I think Rob wants to sleep with other women. Do you think he hates my body because I'm pregnant? Also, *I'm* not that interested in sex."

Has she really heard what I'm saying? Will she hear it only when she says it to another woman?

Do I really believe I'm growing wise with child? *I do.*

June 16, 1978

Sweet baby. You're sick. You have a fever of 101. You're limp, like a dazed and wounded puppy. You've lost your "personality." You haven't enough energy to have a personality.

Babies are invalids: precious elderly souls. They reign in vulnerability. If their screams aren't loud enough to summon assistance, they will die.

Ariel. Little soul.

"But 101 isn't anything for a baby," an experienced mother tells me. "Wait until you see 106 on the thermometer."

June 18, 1978

Your fever's gone. I tiptoe in to look at you: you're awake! Your smile spreads to your eyes. It lights up your nose. You mirror my joy at seeing you well again.

I stay with you as you fall back to sleep. What's this? A flash of silver in your mouth? A beginning tooth!

Ariel: You force me to re-define intimacy. Am I "close" to people with whom I discuss ideas: four times a year? Am I close to friends with whom I can most be myself: by appointment only? Am I close to strangers who thrill me with their decency, wisdom, humor, with whom I don't live?

I'm not as close to anyone as I am to you. And I hardly know you.

Am I grown provincial, tribal, with child? I think so . . .

June 21, 1978

I sit here writing.

"What should I feed him for lunch? You didn't tell me."
My mother is here for the afternoon.

"I have no idea. I'm working now," I say. Still concentrating. "Ask his father. Ask yourself."

"I don't think it's right," she insists. "You're his mother.
You should know what he eats." She stands there waiting.

"Out. Get out," I scream. "You're here to help, not to
house-train me in motherhood. If I were a son, you'd tiptoe
around me not to disturb me."

"I can't understand you. I thought you wanted me here,"
she says. Hurt. Cunningly.

"She has no respect for me or my work," I storm to
your father. *Still refusing to believe what I know is so. Still hoping
it will change.*

How many more times, Mother? How many more times,
before you die, do you *have* to accept me as I am?

How many more times do I have to accept you?

June 24, 1978

They've begun again. (Have they ever stopped?) The moving pictures of your violent death. You fall on your head—and your head splits open. You cough, turn blue before my eyes. One morning you simply don't wake up. You drown in an inch of bath water. You're hit by a car. There's more blood now than when you were born.

I look away. I squeeze my eyes shut.

"David, do you have images of Ariel's death?" I ask.

"All the time," he says.

Death has never frightened me before. Is it because I don't feel as responsible for myself as I do for you, Ariel?

Ariel: Your existence tests my character. Could I abandon you and still consider myself a good person?

Your existence challenges the kind of social contract I've made—or neglected to make. Who will shelter us in storm, whom will we shelter? You force me to deal with the absence of a supportive community in my life. Not for your sake—but for mine. Your coming reminds me of my long-neglected social needs.

June 25, 1978

Ariel, I'd be lying if I romanticized being with you for more than an hour at a time. After fifteen minutes I'm bored with you. But I'm unable to pull myself away.

You are too consuming. *Soft silk.*

You are too limited. *Bashful smile.*

I have other things in my life. *Little belly.*

June 26, 1978

I stand here with other mothers, talking about babies and children. I have never done this before. The world turned upside down.

Everywhere, it seems, women over thirty are having babies. Just at this party, I've found three newborn mothers.

We all want another baby. Why? We can't yet handle the one we have.

Do I "bore"—in not talking about the flow of money, events, men, but in talking about your existence? Each woman's anecdote, every maternal sigh, brings me close to, expresses the religious feelings I have about you. To have this private emotion in public, in chorus, is a little like praying. Social sanctification. The "small talk" of women . . .

"Tough" female voices assail me at prayer.

"There goes Phyllis down the drain. Has a baby, thinks it's the center of *everyone's* life, not just her own. Disgusting, indulgent, self-destructive . . ."

Oh my sisters: Does our mother's flesh so revolt us? Is our female flesh so painful you deny it in the name of woman's survival, woman's freedom?

June 28, 1978

"It's been months since you listened to anything I have to say," I complain to your father.

"You have the nerve to complain I'm not listening to you?" he explodes. "I have no time to listen to you. I'm taking care of a baby! Do you know what that means? I've never worked so hard in my life. The Israeli Army was easier!"

"Why does mothering assume such cosmic proportions when a man does it?" I ask. "World: Stop! Pitch in, offer helpful suggestions. I guess men aren't used to working in utter isolation, as mothers are . . ."

I'm not either. The prospect fills me with horror. Your father is staring at me. Silently.

"Do you want me to applaud you for undertaking 'woman's work'?" I ask him. "Do you applaud me when I pay the bills? You're like a new swimmer splashing too hard in the deep water. You're showing off. And just in case you start drowning, you want everyone to know exactly where you are."

"Why did you want a baby if you won't take care of him?" he asks me.

"Et tu, Brute?" I say.

"What would you do if I walked out?" he whispers. "You couldn't take care of him by yourself."

"You're his father," I yell. "You can't leave. Do you really want him to grow up without being close to a man?"

I hate your father. I love your father. If he consults with me one more time about your diaper rash while I'm working, I may kill your father.

*J*uly 4, 1978

On the beach today, an eight-year-old boy stopped by our blanket.

"Did you see my white butterfly?" he asked.

"No, I haven't," I said. "But in my experience, butterflies are hard to catch."

"Sure. But I'm looking."

Children didn't speak to me before. How do they know that the mother fever's got me? Your satin palms. Your high sweet voice. That body warmth, that toothless smile.

If I feel this way now, how will I feel when you can ask me about butterflies?

July 5, 1978

We took you to the movies last night—never again! Suddenly, you started crying. I thought I'd die. *I thought they'd kill me.* Your father quieted you with a bottle. I held you in the dark: rigid, frightened.

The second time you howled, I went through the floor and ceiling simultaneously.

"Hey, lady. Get that kid out of here."

"Take him home. Shut him up."

Where are the people who tell me I can take you everywhere? Did anyone ever stone women for noisy babies? If not, why so intense a reaction on my part?

July 6, 1978

Moving you from the house to the beach is like moving a small army. There's your bottle of water, and one of formula to prepare. There's fruit to mash and put in a container. There are diapers and towelettes to count and ointment to pack. An umbrella for your blond skin. A car seat for you to sit on in the sand. A special terry towel. A sweater. Have I forgotten anything? I check again. By the time I've packed everything, I'm cranky. And it's time to feed or change you. Or you're sleeping.

How do other parents manage?

July 10, 1978

Nobody loves you when you're down and out. Newly rich people have no real friends.

To be a mother is to be newly rich *and* down and out.

As long as I pass for being single or child-free; as long as I hide my sense of being crushed by (un)natural responsibility; as long as I remain well-mannered in public—I remain acceptable.

For how long? What if I started crying? What if I made too many personal demands?

Hello, Nora, Sharon, Carolyn: I'm lonely, isolated. I feel my life has ended. I'm stuck at home. Please come over and play with me. Or invite us all over for dinner. I'll never trust any of you again if you don't . . .

Hello, Miriam, Suzanne, Pamela: I want you to move next door. I need to see you casually, spontaneously. Our friendship feels like a gift, reward! I want family feeling between us instead. If we can't have that, I'll . . . what? Kill myself? Kill you? Threaten, silently, to put all my love into you, Ariel, withdraw it from the world?

Who'd care? Women, men, do just that with every child.

July 12, 1978

Your father leaps up at your slightest cry. He makes me feel useless, incompetent. He says I'm not as good with you as he is. He tells other people so.

Is this how "fathers" are traditionally made to feel by "mothers"? Well-meaning, but only suited for paying the bills. "Fathers": thrown over for an infant. Ariel: What guilt, what rage I feel about not being your most preferred parent.

I'm not worried. If I don't like what's happening, I can: *(a)* run away; *(b)* run away with you; *(c)* ask your father to please throw himself out the window; or *(d)* bribe your father to run away with you. I have other possibilities too. There's always *(e)* taking a wife or *(f)* not caring. How can I not care?

Ariel: You keep me honest. The minute I make a wild pronouncement, if I don't really mean it, I'm the first to take it back.

July 15, 1978

After six months of motherhood, I understand that taking care of what needs to be done, from day to day, is all there is. I can't plan too far in advance.

This makes everything both easier and harder: easier because I can reduce my standards for myself to daily ones. Harder because no matter what I do, it will never be enough. There is always another day.

That mother's complaint.

July 20, 1978

Suddenly I find myself thinking about my mother. How is she? What is she doing? I pick up the phone to find out. *I feel close to her for the first time in my life.*

I can't be like my mother. I can't allow myself to be swallowed up by either the experience or the institution of motherhood. My mother's behavior shows me, too clearly, the horrible price it exacted of her.

I feel close to my mother. . . . No. Becoming a mother somehow allows me to admit, to act on, what I've always felt: *my love for her.*

This is incredible! *I love my mother.* I've never said this to her. She's never said this to me. We're not friends. We don't have a "good" time together.

Our conversations are thick with innuendo and unspoken desire. We know how to say what we're expected to say, how to avoid saying that which must not be said. *I love you. I need you.* I love her because she is my mother. She loves me—now I am certain of it—because I am her daughter. Until now this has not been sufficient. It becomes more so.

She knows too much. She keeps asking me how often I feed you by myself. How often I change you by myself. I know what she's getting at. I don't like it, but it makes me laugh. She knows that I don't do these things as much as she did. She won't rest until she gets me to be more like her.

Between mother and daughter there is no middle point. There is All or Nothing.

July 22, 1978

Today I swung you up and, together, we faced your favorite person—yourself—in the mirror.

"Ariel," I chided. "I have always looked for myself. Maybe I've found her in you. Are you already in search of yourself too?"

I have found myself and left myself behind in each of my books. Will we leave each other behind too? With this pregnancy, I thee wed. With this birth, I sever our flesh bond forever.

July 24, 1978

Ariel: Today I didn't leave town because I couldn't leave you. Am I in love with you? *I spent two hours staring into your eyes.* And I didn't go out last night. I manufactured a headache—I lied!—in order to be with you. I didn't say: "I'm canceling my obligation because I prefer being with my son." How could I say that?

Sweet baby! Your teeth are bothering you terribly. How can I leave you?

Dancing with you, kissing you, is romantic. You feel like all the Prince Valiants I've ever dreamed of, like the darkest of lovers, in blond.

Last night, as I played with you, my womb began to ache with desire for another child. How much more I would romanticize a pregnancy now.

We can't afford another baby.

July 28, 1978

"Mother-thinking": If I write a book about you, and you die, it's because I wrote the book.

"Mother-thinking": If I do something *just for me* for a whole afternoon, and you die, it's because I put myself first.

"Mother-thinking": If I go out with friends and leave you with a baby-sitter, and you die, it's my fault. It would never have happened if I had been home, "where I belong."

The belief that a mother is powerful enough to prevent death. The belief that "trade-offs" can be made: my life for my child's.

Even the Virgin Mary couldn't do it.

To glorify such delusions of omnipotence! To be silenced or ostracized *by other women* if you admit maternal powerlessness.

"Mother-guilt": The reverse of delusions of maternal omnipotence.

My friend Angie, a mother of three, *doesn't* have delusions of omnipotence.

"But," she reminds me, "my mother won't talk to me. My mother can't deal with my being divorced. She hates the fact that I *wanted* joint custody. She despises me for working. She thinks I should be home with the kids all the time, at least until the youngest is fifteen. That's eleven years from now. If I did that, I'd probably be too afraid to ever leave the house. Like my mother is."

"It's unbelievable," I respond. "But my mother thinks like that too. My upstairs and downstairs neighbors, both new mothers, think this way. The law courts think this way. And horrible to say, it's an advance of sorts. Once, women were thought to have no souls. Only fathers could shape children's characters, mold children's behavior. Mothers? Good for suckling, mending, cooking."

"Phyllis," she tells me, "don't pay attention to any mother who tells you to stay home, as she did. Ask her if she'll watch your kid, since she's so big on it. And you're not."

*A*ugust 4, 1978

In bed with you. Forbidden pleasures. Tongue in tongue, wetly, laughing. Sucking, licking, stroking. Eyes shut: mine. Eyes impassively open: yours. Your eyes close only when you thrust your thumb deeply into your mouth, grab a tiny handful of my hair, move it close, and become one with me, one with yourself, sucking fiercely, steadily, again. Your passion.

Ariel, you've come between your parents. You're a Home-Wrecker, more dangerous than a thousand Helens of Troy. We must choose: you—or each other. We choose you. *Your father* chooses to be with you, not with me.

I dare not complain: Who would listen? Who would be sympathetic? I'm the jealous one. I want you all to myself. I want David all to myself. I don't want to share either of you.

I'm the child—not you, Ariel: You teach me about myself, about my imperfections, every day. Sweet teacher.

August 8, 1978

A divorced mother is telling me how she lost custody of her children.

"First, their father stopped making love to me. He humiliated me in the bedroom. He ran in first when the baby cried. He diapered her faster. He pointed this out to all our relatives. Laughing. He made a big deal of relating to the children altogether. The whole neighborhood said: What a wonderful father! What a lucky mother! Then he stole my babies away from me legally! Everyone helped him. This is exactly what happened to me."

A cold wind blows across my back.

"But don't you think it's crucial for fathers to get involved in parenting? . . . "

"Yeah, but they take over, they "do it better." They compete with you for your children's love. You begin to feel incompetent, guilty. You get angry at your kids for not seeing through his trick. For not automatically loving you more. Why should I have to compete for my children's love?

"Then their father criticized my cooking. He didn't like how the kids were dressed. He sent his mother over to watch me while he wasn't home. Everyone started talking.

"When I went for a divorce, *my mother and sisters* testified against me. How could I be a good mother if I want a divorce?

" 'Stay married,' they yelled at me.

" 'No more,' I screamed back.

"So I lost my little babies. Their father has them. Every day he turns them against me more. They don't look me in the eye when I manage to arrange a visit. Which isn't often. By the time they're grown up, they'll hate me or not care one way or the other. He's got them.

"He owns them. He doesn't have to be so 'good' anymore. He has his mother and a new wife for the kids. He can go back to being the father: high and mighty."

She sits forward. Intent.

"No mother is safe from this happening. The courts will give the children to the fathers—and send us on welfare or into mental asylums. Maybe they'll allow us to work as secretaries, salesgirls—teachers, if I finish my special classes. Nothing that will ever give me enough money. Nothing as precious to me as my kids were."

Ariel: She's warned me. What if your father decides that his "maternal" responsibility to you equals exclusive legal ownership? That my not diapering you as often as he does makes me a "bad mother"? What if he decides to punish me because he doesn't really want to take care of you—by doing it and then using it as the excuse for taking you away?

Your pediatrician will say that your father, not your mother, brought you for your checkups. The baby-sitters can testify that your father, not your mother, watched them, criticized them, "cared" more about what they did for you than I did.

My own mother doesn't like our child care arrangement. What would a male judge think of it?

Where can I run with you? If I did, I'd still have to hire a housekeeper to care for you. I'd have to work very hard to pay her salary. I could still be accused of being a "bad mother." I could lose you—unless I were protected by a very wealthy and powerful family. Which I'm not. (Who is?)

Mothers don't accuse men of being "bad fathers" if they're not home all the time. Maybe fathers should stand accused. But who would support the children, if women can't earn enough money—as mothers, or as anything else?

The tender trap.

Woe, women!

When *we* mother, we're valued poorly, and worked like slaves. No matter how efficient we are, our children can be taken away from us by their fathers. *If they're bent on it.* We can easily be abandoned, without emotional or economic support for ourselves or our children. Without a respectable and direct wage for mothering.

When *we* work "outside the home," we're ostracized and paid too little money. We're not seen as heroines breaking barriers, or as mothers feeding ourselves and families, but as ball-busters who have to be stopped. Or as drones, there to be used. We're pitied: for not having found men to buy us at a high enough price.

August 12, 1978

"I'm still breast-feeding at night," Stephanie tells me. "But the pediatrician yelled at me. He said I was making love to my daughter. That it was disgusting, dangerous."

"What!" I yell.

"Well, she's two years old. What if he's right? What if I'm doing it more for me than for her? I've been depressed ever since I saw him. Even though I disagree with him. I hate him for making me feel guilty."

"Stephanie, I wish I were still breast-feeding. I only stopped because I had to go on the road for three months. I know breast-feeding is exhausting and ties you down. But how can it be bad for a baby? Maybe it's bad for you."

"No one is worrying about what's bad for me. The doctor thinks I like it too much. He doesn't believe that my daughter likes it even more!"

"Stephanie, if you want to wean, it should be because *you* need to. Because *you're* too tired or too busy. I can't imagine how breast-feeding at night is bad for a two-year-old!"

But the doctors think it is. Stephanie described two physicians, male and female: supercilious, pitying. Angry. Can they possibly envy the baby her mother's milk? The woman her pleasure?

*A*ugust 14, 1978

Phantom kicks in my womb! Wonderful, strange. The body never forgets. *My* body never will forget *you*. Sometimes I can still squeeze milk out of my nipples. Especially when I'm wearing one of my January or February dressing gowns. Especially when tenderness floods through me as I look at you. If we had to, could I sustain you with it?

You are spun out of silk, spun out of satin.

We've raised the bar on the crib. You look as if you're in a cage. You're a prisoner of our needs, of our limitations.

August 21, 1978

Ariel: When I hold you close, I feel us as One. I'm comforted by having you near. Strange, that I didn't feel "at one" with myself when I was pregnant.

Why such comfort now that you're outside?

Where shall we live, little one? Where do single-income middle-class families go? Into exile in suburbia, where dusk pierces my heart with loneliness?

I don't want to live too far from your grandmother. I'd like us to have dinner with her once a week. You make me want again what I've always wanted, never had: family life.

The Hallmark-greeting-card dybbuk has got me. I dream of family portraits and heirlooms. Hot cocoa, ice skating, red-cheeked holidays.

*A*ugust 24, 1978

In bed with you alone: you touch my palm more expertly than any earthly lover. I moan with pleasure. You fidget, startle, become "only" a baby.

Ariel: I must talk to you. I'm afraid of what I've done. Summoning you into this world when I need a mother myself.

Ariel: Where will you live in the next century? What if the flames of human cruelty and ignorance are more hideous than I can imagine? Will you flee across the face of famine, war, disease, looking for me? *Where am I?* Will you find me? Will it help?

Will you at least have your youth? Only that: no more?

Who else will love you? Whom will you love?

I'll be seventy-five years old when you're my age.

*A*ugust 26, 1978

Colette's mother, Sido, said to her daughter: "Now you're a *writer* who gave birth to a child."

Yes. Never will I be a "mother first" or a "mother only." How strange that I regret that this is so. *I would like to be able to drown in you, Ariel. Safely. Just for a year or two. Not for a lifetime. I crave Dionysius rising. Apollo rules me still.*

You've exposed my habit, my craving for order, meaning. How tenaciously I cling to it. Even against you. Oh, if I only could "let go," give up, drop out.

I can't.

*A*ugust 31, 1978

Death. Poverty. Illness. No room of one's own. Illiteracy. Fatigue. *An utter lack of encouragement.* Each, all, have silenced women before on the subject of pregnancy and motherhood.

One editor, sharp-tongued, fast-moving, tells me that the subject of motherhood doesn't turn her on—her phrase.

"You should write meatier stuff for me, something a person can really sink her teeth into. Theoretical stuff. Political stuff."

I say nothing. I don't believe what I've just heard.

A second editor yells at me. "What kind of example do you mean to set? Are you trying to convince women to return to their cages willingly?" she asks. "Biological reproduction has been the downfall of women."

Silence deepens within me. Fear. Disbelief.

"What I'd really like from you, Phyllis," a third editor confides, "is a novel. Something gorgeous, commercial. Anyone can write about motherhood. It's been done."

They don't ask to read anything: *an utter lack of encouragement.*

One editor who wants this journal can't acquire it.

"Phyllis, I'm so sorry," she says. "My boss just went crazy. He yelled and screamed about your other books. *He said he didn't like it that you have a child.* He said whatever you write couldn't possibly represent the true feelings of women about motherhood. . . . "

Ariel: I wonder how long I can continue to write: this diary, or anything else. The money is never enough to live on. How long before I retire to a chicken farm, to a counting house, into silence? How long before I, too, start to write "on the side"?

September 1, 1978

Here's what I feel, after four months at home with you:
Mothers are good for one thing—making others comfortable.
Don't plot too ambitious a course for yourself. Don't call
too much attention to your distress or anger. Things could
be worse. Don't blame anyone but yourself.

Stick to your pots, woman. Bend your head to the babe.
Leave the rest to the wealthy, and to those with no children.
Smile an awful lot. Your fate is in the hands of others.

Here's a ten-year prescription for Valium. Renewable
for ten years more. The liquor store is two blocks away,
bakeries are everywhere. A color television set: your daily
companion. Escape novels: imagine being raped by a prince
and loving it in every century. Imagine being someone else.
Imagine that you're dead.

Are there any questions? O.K., ladies. Forward march.

September 3, 1978

Our new schedule: From 7 A.M. to 4 P.M. every day, you're in your father's keeping. When he's in school, from 5 to 10 P.M. four nights a week, I have you. Weekends, we share you.

From 8 to 4 every day, I write in this diary, work on a radio column, answer my mail, return phone calls. I write and deliver one lecture a month. I also read manuscripts, make referrals, do consultations, give interviews, oversee research for another book, and turn up, breathlessly, at professional meetings. *Sometimes I even meet a friend for lunch.*

I see patients, "paying guests," for a few hours each day, and for one long evening every week.

I never have time to rest. Neither does David. We are both always working.

Late afternoon is my treasure time. But just as I'm about to give you a five-minute kiss, your father appears with tea for both of us. Sometimes you fall asleep just as I come on duty. The phone keeps ringing. My assistant runs in to check something with me.

We're constantly surrounded by other people. I'd like to spirit you away—but how?

When it's Merri's night to baby-sit, she bursts in to hug both of us. "Phyllis," she says, "I feel I'm becoming part of the family."

"Oh, you are. Yes," I affirm. "It's been going on since we met last January."

"I'd like to baby-sit for Ariel three nights a week," she says. "I love to be with him. I think of it as a feminist thing to do: to make it more possible for you to survive."

I'm stunned. I can scarcely believe it. Someone is offering to do something personally to help *me.* In a spirit of sisterhood.

My apprentice, my daughter, my sister. Is this what they mean when they say babies bring their own luck?

September 4, 1978

Never, never, could *I* have felt close to my mother without becoming a mother too. Never before could I get past my hot rage at her cruelty to me. Did I need to be overwhelmed by the demands of motherhood before I could soften, even slightly, toward her? Is it she who's softened?

I tend to over-romanticize her. I can't help it. She, and you, are genuinely romantic happenings in my life.

Still, I'm afraid a Bad Mother—mine—reigns inside me. House-trapped. Resigned. Cold. Disorganized. Whenever I'm home with you alone, that's how I feel. When I'm away from you, I feel like my "old" self: competent, energetic.

So much is the process of sustaining life devalued, I experience it as dangerous, negative.

So valued is adult, child-less activity, I experience it as bright, redeeming.

September 5, 1978

The park: a sandbox, swings, a semicircle of benches. I can *see* the trees. My blurred universe slows down, assumes color, becomes precise. Remembrances of things past.

You, a child, do this. Like madeleine cakes, you fill me with memories. Perceptions of my own childhood.

"What a lovely child!" a woman said today, watching you play.

"Yes, he is wonderful, isn't he!" I replied, in wonder.

I've heard mothers say "thank you" when their child is complimented. I don't. How can I take credit for your sweetness, your beauty, your precious sense of humor? You are your own miracle.

September 11, 1978

My respect for women as mothers deepens. I'm frightened when heroines are so insecure, so guilty. One mother, speaking slowly, tells me:

"I can blame my husband all I want. And it's true: When he lived with us, emotions were rationed, feelings frozen. It's much better now that he's moved out. But I still know that inside me is something so monstrous, so powerful, it could kill my children. It could poison them slowly. My bitterness. My anger."

Mine too, Sister.

Muriel, a mother of grown-up children, confirms the isolation of motherhood for me.

"It's real. But there's something worse. A child can hurt you more than anyone else ever could. And then walk away, forget it. The pain stays with *you* almost forever. . . . Now, that's true of the joys too. No one can make you as happy as a child."

"Who helped you with your children?" I ask her.

"My mother, of course. Who else can you count on?"

"Phyllis," Mary tells me, "you never stop being a mother. My daughter is twenty-one and we can't cut the cord."

I feel expansive.

"Mary," I joke, "even in the army, you get a furlough, you get a discharge. Are you saying that mothers are on sentry duty forever?"

"Yes, ma'am. There's no way I can stop feeling responsible for her."

September 13, 1978

We've just interviewed our third male applicant as a part-time baby-sitter.

"I'm very neat," this one says. "I'm very quiet."

"What do you do when you're not working?" your father asks him.

"Oh, I sleep. I watch television. I don't have friends. Who can you trust these days?"

"What were you doing for the last year?" I ask.

"I was valet for a single gentleman."

"He's not gay," I tell your father afterward. "He's an ex-inmate of some mental asylum."

"You discriminate against ex-crazies?" your father jokes with me. "Maybe you don't like him because he's a man?"

"He's the weirdest of the lot. . . . I sense enormous violence in him," I say.

"Me too." Your father agrees. "How suspicious we both are of a man wanting this job. Is this how men feel about women in engineering or plumbing?"

"Not a fair comparison," I say. "The women applying there are usually *better* than most men. They have to be. These male would-be housekeepers are all underqualified. They're rejecting "men's work," and they don't seem to know the first thing about "women's work." At best, they're fit to care for the clothes and food of a bachelor colonel. What do they know about running a household and caring for a baby, the way a woman does?"

Ariel: I'll be honest. I don't want this man near you. His frustration tolerance is too low. I fear he's incompetent, violent.

Ariel: I'm not saying *you're* like this. But you might be, if you don't have gentle, loving men surrounding you. Besides your father, where can we find such men: for hire?

September 15, 1978

How long the weekends are! Before you, a weekend was the collapsible-expandable part of the week. I collapsed down into it and when I got up, the weekend was gone. Or weekends expanded into long, uninterrupted work weeks.

A weekend now is All Ariel. Friday night, Saturday, Sunday: inelastic, forbidding. Each has a morning, an afternoon, a late afternoon, an early evening, a late evening, and a whole night through.

Every one of these time sections must be covered if I want to be "off duty." That means arranging something beforehand: with your father, your grandmother, with Merri, with baby-sitters.

September 20, 1978

Today is my mother's birthday. Can anyone ever replace her in my life? Can anyone else ever give birth to me? I am one of those women who's found part of the mother I never had, or lost, in a husband.

Today I wonder about this. Does your coming couple us forever? Must I always live with your father for your sake? Or for my sake, because no one will care as much about you, besides me, as he does? *What if my mother wanted me back?* Are we tied, then, your father and I, against our will? For convenience, out of fear? Will I break and run because of this? Will I test this tie over and over again, to make sure it won't break?

What if it does? What if it doesn't?

Can't we all three live under the same roof, but in separate apartments? Can't we live as friendly Buddhist monks, sacredly tied, but separate, separate? I feel more cramped now than I did this time last year.

Happy birthday, Mother. If you hadn't been born, there would be no Ariel.

September 23, 1978

I asked a Mother what she thinks a "good mother" is.

"A good mother is nothing like me," she said. "A good mother always knows what to do, and does it well, without complaining, without yelling, without manipulating anyone. A good mother uses her power to protect her children from all harm. A good mother has healthy, happy, wonderful children. A good mother is nothing like my mother, or like my grandmother. . . ."

"You're describing a faery goddess and a machine," I interrupt.

"Yes, maybe I am. But I think that's what a good mother should be."

September 25, 1978

Last night the mother of a twenty-year-old took me aside.

"I think it's harder when they're older," she whispered. "You don't know where they are. They don't listen to you. And you can't stop yourself from worrying. At Ariel's age, well, there he is. Always with you. Loving you right back."

Another mother says, darkly:

"Enjoy that baby while you still can. Later on, forget it. They break everything. Then they buy everything. Then they're gone. Forever."

I have been gone from my mother. Forever.

September 27, 1978

You're crying. I'm fighting with your father. The phone keeps ringing. We're out of diapers. Everyone's laundry is undone. I haven't a single pair of underpants to wear. I'm late for a meeting.

I understand what makes mothers run away. I understand what happens when mothers stay. Colored gray. Colored irritable.

I don't want to live my childhood over again. I don't want to be my mother: trapped. I don't want to grow so bitter that you'll never know me as a "laughing girl," except from old photographs taken before you were born.

For your sake, for my sake, I want to avoid even one more day like today.

How? Today I asked my mother to come over and help.

"I can't," she said. "Don't count on me," she said. For the eightieth time.

Why do I keep asking her? Who else can I ask?

Last week I met a new mother together with *her* mother in the park. The young mother looked gray. She babbled. She apologized for each sentence.

"Do you get any time off?" I asked her.

"Of course not," the grandmother, robust, healthy, answered. "She's a breast-feeding mother. What could be more important than her being with my lovely grandson?"

"Do you help her?" I ask point-blank.

"Help? She doesn't need my help. What kind of help do you mean?" The grandmother looks menacing.

"No, no, I'm O.K.," the mother whispers. "It's only been six months without sleep. When he sleeps through the night, everything will be fine. Really fine." Her eyes look downward, inward.

A "good daughter" is a woman who "dies" in child birth, like her mother before her.

I'm not a "good daughter." I'm not a "good mother." I won't go down without a fight. *Whom do I have to fight?* You? Your father? My mother? All patriarchy? Life itself?

No, not life. Something is wrong if new mothers turn gray, idiotic. Turn silent. Something is wrong with a culture that considers new mothers so expendable.

Why can't this gray mother turn to her mother for help? Why aren't there good child care centers on every corner? Outreach programs for new parents in every neighborhood? Check-ups for mothers right after childbirth—and regularly afterwards? Something's wrong with my lower back. . . .

September 28, 1978

Risa and I, in the evening rain, talking motherhood.

"Risa," I ask, "did you ever really love anyone before your son?"

"No, I never did," she says. "That's why I can't live with his father now. I can't bear the unreality between us. Compared to what I know is possible with my child."

"I've let Ariel teach me lessons about life that I've refused to learn elsewhere," I tell her.

"Oh, yes. Motherhood can do that. But not if you're cooped up day and night alone with your child. Every mother I know in Israel, including me, is a *working* mother. It's no big deal. Everyone knows that a child will be watched by her mother, her father, by relatives, by a private housekeeper *and* by a government employee in a child care center."

"It sounds unreal," I say.

"I drop my son off at the governess's house at ten every morning. I pick him up at four in the afternoon. Fifteen little children in the courtyard wave bye-bye to him when we leave. And he's only two years old! He's always smiling, curious."

"What do you do in the evenings about baby-sitting?" I ask.

"I have a long list of baby-sitters for the evening. I have a neighbor with children. Sometimes we exchange evenings out."

"It's not like that for me here," I say. Holding my breath in anger and sorrow. "I know very few new mothers who are my age, or who have commitments outside the home like I do. I'm lonely."

"It's *crazy* here," she whispers. "The mothers isolated from each other—still. Not working because they have a baby. Trapped indoors in the cold weather. And can you believe? They think it's better for the child this way?"

Sweet, sweet words! "Risa, why don't you call my mother up and explain all this to her?" I laugh.

"Mother trouble? I'm not very close to mine. She doesn't know where she ends and I start."

"No. No mother trouble. We're reconciled. Now that we're both mothers. It's just that she thinks I should stay home full-time with Ariel."

"You're joking," Risa says.

I wish I were.

September 29, 1978

"Better go on a crash diet, Phyllis. Can't you get away for a month to a health spa?"

Donna looks at her own gently potted stomach with disgust.

"Come with me," she suggests. "I have to lose five pounds."

Are biological mothers supposed to pass for non-mothers? How many women make love in the dark, or not at all, because of stretch marks? Because we no longer look eighteen?

Warrior marks. Natural signposts of human experience. My breasts are round, resigned. I'm fat. My flesh is abnormally soft.

Where is my young girl hiding? The one with all the angles: in her voice, in her breasts?

Did she leave me when I became a Mother?

September 30, 1978

You suck your bottle. Large trustful eyes over your sucking mouth. Watching me watch you.

What do you see? A Lady in coffee? A Mother?

It took this long for me to realize that I missed menstruating when I was pregnant.

How long will it take me to remember, to appreciate *this* moment?

Psychic communication exists between us. We don't have to reach each other through words. I don't speak slowly, loudly, as if you speak another language. We *both* speak that other language: of knowing, of being.

Ariel: I always say I went back to work for days after you were born. The truth is, I've stuck to the house like glue. Working, yes: *but at home.* Near you.

We've only been apart against my will. Even now, with all the noise you make, I can't bring myself to rent a separate studio. Not yet.

October 1, 1978

I hear my mother speaking.

"Grow up," she says. Gently. "Put yourself second. Overlook the slights, the difficulties. Nothing is black or white. There is only gray."

"I can't put myself second. It's too painful."

"You will. You're a mother now."

"I didn't decide to give up my work or my sanity in order to have a baby. Ariel has a father—and a grandmother too. . . ."

"But you're his mother. Don't you *want* to spend all your time with him? He's so precious."

"No. I'd like to spend *more* time. Not all my time. Anyway, mothers get blamed no matter how hard they try. Mothers aren't respected. . . .*I* haven't respected you."

She smiles. Keeps silent.

I'm feeling her power—strongly—without fighting about it. Without running from it. Without feeling humiliated by it. I'm hearing her talk about her religion: motherhood. Not *my* religion, but worthy of my respect.

She's tired. She's puzzled by my wanting to talk to her so much. She sighs.

"You have to accept your children as they are."

"Why? You don't accept me as I am. You're always trying to change me," I remind her. Gently.

She smiles again. "I keep hoping. I haven't totally given up on you. You're still my child too."

"You expect much more of me than of my brothers. . . ."

"You're my eldest. You're a mother. And you're still a baby."

Mother: How can you be a diplomat among your children *and* also their chambermaid, without going crazy? The street cleaner who whispers into the emperor's ear? The woman who says the emperor is naked? The woman who remains silent?

Mother: You run from child to child, whispering peace, whispering "My way," as if each child is a country, with boundaries only you can cross. You serve each country its meals, do its laundry. With a turned back, you incite guilt. With harsh words, anger and sorrow. Such a tyrannical servant!

Mother: What do you do when the children all unite against you? Who comforts you then?

Today is my thirty-eighth birthday.

October 3, 1978

Standing in the rain, waiting for you to arrive with your father. Another mother stands with me, waiting for a glimpse of you.

"Lois," I ask, "what do you do when it doesn't feel worthwhile and you can't run away and you can't cope either?"

"Double martini," she says cheerfully. "Vitamins are important too. If you don't keep yourself in good health, forget it!"

She's wonderfully matter-of-fact.

"Here's what mothers need, Phyllis: Maids. Baby-sitters. Lots of space. Money. And don't stay home. Work outside. Come and go. Linger, and you die, bit by bit. I love my kids, but I never found them interesting as infants, or as young children."

"Why did you become a mother?" I ask.

"We're talking about thirty years ago. The first one was an accident. The second was to keep him company. The third just happened."

"Who helped you out?"

"Never have a baby without a good husband and a good grandmother."

Two women are smiling in the rain. And here you are, all blond and serious and very late.

"Oh, he's worth it," Lois says. "Doesn't look like you, does he?"

October 5, 1978

Ariel: Your father has taken care of you for the last six months. Now he says it's too much, he can't *study* and be a mother. Your coming has galvanized him into taking himself seriously.

But where does this leave you? Fatherless like all the other children! Soon, soon, he'll be absent from your daily life: enough for you to begin to fear and idealize him—and after him, all men.

You too, sweet one, will be brought up essentially by women. By me: and by all the women I can afford to hire.

Where, now, is our society's fabled love of motherhood and children? Where are the foundation and government grants for *personal* child care? Where are the well-paying part-time jobs for parents?

I don't want to work so hard that I'm tired and irritable when I'm with you.

I don't want to work so many hours that I have no time for myself apart from you.

I don't want to give literally everything I earn to house-keepers, baby-sitters, secretaries. I don't want to keep working only to earn money—or only so that I'm allowed to keep working.

I don't want to "drop out" for five years to be with you full-time. *That* would drive me as mad as what we have now.'

Child: I grieve. I storm. A lump of disbelief and a lump of bitterness grow small and hard in me. They are my two pupils, looking out at the world.

October 10, 1978

You squeeze the rubber ball, squeaking it. You grow insane with triumph. You clench your teeth. Your excitement is unbearable. In your eyes, a wild gleam of fear. You rock unsteadily on your feet, squeaking away. Drunk with power.

My tiny watchman of the crib. You check each corner, every toy, make certain everything is there. After you've made your rounds, you fall asleep at the center, watched over by your bear, your camel, your mobile. Watched over by me.

Ariel: Will you have children? Will they look like me? Will you see me in one of them? Why am I thinking about this?

What if you're the only fruit of my father's flight from Poland? My mother's only grandchild?

*O*ctober 14, 1978

Drawing close to the child in me, I move easily between extremes of emotion. I'm learning to forget one moment as I enter another moment. I'm becoming ruthless in the way I spend my being-time. I have no time, no energy, for anything non-essential. I leave places quickly when I'm bored.

To rush home to you. Tonight I was downtown listening to chamber music "for a worthy cause." Windows cut into white brick walls soared to double-height ceilings. The moon rose in one window. A tree branch fluttered in another. The kitchen gleamed like a sculpture by Judy Chicago. People sampled dips, inclined their heads to the original music.

I run down the stairs, run to find a cab, hesitate: should I go to a movie now that I'm out, alone and free?

"Uptown," I tell the driver. I want to be with you. I'll surprise you. Are you still up? I sit in the back seat like a teen-ager in love.

You're awake! What screams of joy. Smiles. We renew our acquaintance every five minutes. Making sure the other is really here, exclaiming our pleasure that we are. Oh, we are.

October 16, 1978

Ariel: Your father baby-sat for another woman's child so she could have some time for herself. Afterward he mentioned it to me—apologetically, as if he thought I'd disapprove.

"She had no time alone since she gave birth," he explains. "Her husband won't help. She looked pretty bad."

I am moved to tears. I have never done this for another mother.

October 18, 1978

"What is your mother like?" a friend asks.

"Comfortable only when she's nursing a slightly—very slightly—sick child. Dimmed lights. Hot tea. Hushed footsteps. A perpetual vigil against germs, disease, the evil eye. My mother is a mother-warrior."

"What does she say, first thing, when she sees you now?"

" 'How can you bear to be away from your baby?' she says at the door. 'I don't understand you! Never have. Never mind. I don't like the way Ariel's eye looks. You've got to take him to a specialist. . . . Look what I found in my closet. Is it yours? What do you want me to do with it?'

"Then she follows me from room to room, gives me newspaper coupons, warnings. She stands outside the closed bathroom door with more questions."

"Is she pretty?"

"Her skin is beautiful: unflawed, unlined, clear. Her eyes are dark. She's slender, small-breasted. Graceful."

Ariel: I love your grandmother.

*O*ctober 22, 1978

This morning my mother asked me if I agreed with the "experts" that mothers should be blamed for everything. Stunned, I tell her how strongly I disagree with this nonsense.

"Oh, you've changed your mind since you became a mother!" She laughs.

"*No. No.*" I run for my 1971 and 1972 lectures about mothers. I read aloud to her.

She listens. She stirs her tea. She *smiles.*

"I told your father I wouldn't read any books on child raising. I'd do it better on my own, I told him. Every time you did something bad, he'd laugh at me, tell me to check into the books. But I didn't. How could a book know my own child?"

I ask her what she wanted to teach me.

"To be smart. To be understanding. To be good. To be healthy."

"I am all that you wanted," I tell her. Earnestly. *Wanting to please her.*

"No. You're not. You should be taking care of Ariel by yourself. All the time. How else can you know him, or teach him to be what you believe in?"

"Careful now," I note. "You're criticizing a mother." Ah, your daughter's a mother too, I crow. Checkmate. In your game, Mother, there are two queens. And we both get to win: each other, immortality.

October 28, 1978

Through you, Ariel, I'm enlarged, connected to something larger than myself. Like falling in love, like ideological conversion, the connection makes me *feel* my existence.

You draw me close to the young girl, the child in me: closer to her than I've been since when?—1945, the year of atomic bombs and block parties? 1952, crinolines and McCarthy hearings?

I'm in California now, *writing* about you. I didn't want to leave you—not for your sake, but for mine. What if my plane crashed and I became childless?

Just as I boarded the plane, you noticed me, screamed your goodbye—and waved.

October 29, 1978

Changing. For example, I no longer defend or even present my beliefs to everyone I meet. When people speak to me in 1950s voices, I listen. I disarm by being as personal as possible.

Last night a man with a depressed wife-in-tow demanded, good-naturedly:

"What will the Equal Rights Amendment really do for women? If *mothers* need to stay at home with children, then isn't ERA irrelevant for most women? Do women like you need the ERA?"

Laughing, I tell him:

"Five days after my child was born, I was working. I *had* to. I'm self-employed. I work at home, and my business needed me as much as my baby did. And yes: women like me need the ERA."

"But be honest," he continues. "Who stays home if your child gets sick—you or your husband?"

"In my particular case, both of us. But when *your* child is sick, aren't you distracted, restless, at work? Don't you call home a lot, try to get there earlier than usual? Wouldn't *you* be at a hospital if your child was in it, no matter what kind of deal you had cooking?"

"Yes, yes," he agrees, no longer in charge of making a "point." Neither am I.

We talk for half an hour. Before you, baby, I couldn't have felt any connection with such a man.

Am I even slightly connected to this man because we have children? Because late at night, talking, we both feel protective of life in a personal way? The implications of this are staggering. People without children move too fast, overturn too much, care too little about conserving life. . . . Ten months ago, I was a person without a child. Was I like that?

Are children the reason we have as much peace on earth as we do?

Are children the cause of war? Forcing parents into looking the other way when it happens? Into joining it if it's "good" for the children?

Are war-makers ever practicing parents?

November 2, 1978

"Coming out" as a mother: what a liberation movement that would be!

A mother, here in California, described her dreams during pregnancy as "strange and vivid."

"But no one would listen to me recount them. Other pregnant women had their own interests. New mothers were sucked up by their babies. Non-mothers couldn't relate. Or I couldn't relate to them. I finally stopped trying to talk. I became quiet," she told me.

Another mother: "After I gave birth, I could only talk to other mothers. But I was afraid to tell them the real truth. So I couldn't trust what they said either."

"What was the 'real truth'?" I asked.

"The loneliness. The isolation. How incompetent I was as a mother. My anger."

"The usual," I say. Relieved to hear it again from another woman.

"But I had no one," she whispers. "I was totally alone. I was afraid I'd hate my baby. I knew I was going to be a bad mother."

November 5, 1978

Since I gave birth, the colors I look good in have changed. I've moved into turquoise, green, blue: the colors of the sea. My rusts and browns hang unchosen in the closet. I've moved off earth into deep waters.

I dress myself in original shades of amniotic fluid.

When I enter your room, especially mornings, the smell of warm, fresh urine, the smell of Desitin, are totally erotic. Before you existed, could I even have tolerated such smells?

November 10, 1978

"I hear you're writing about childbirth," Irene says. "Good, it's time. I wish I could have. No one would have published it. Not then."

"When did you give birth?" I ask.

"During World War Two, in New York City. It was a battleground. Women crowded together in corridors, in rooms. All in labor. None of us instructed by anyone about anything. You can't imagine. The horror of watching other women giving birth—the amount of blood—as you were in pain yourself.

"A very young girl was strapped down on a gurney. Her eyes were wheeling around in fear. A doctor examined her. Roughly, loudly, he said, 'Just my goddamn luck to get a breech birth.' And he walked away. No comforting. No explaining."

"A battleground. Warriors without medals," I comment.

Irene laughs. "That's a wonderful idea! But things have changed since then—haven't they?"

"I don't think so. Not for most women in America. With all my book information; with all my professional knowledge of hospitals and experts; with a friendly obstetrician of my choice; with a midwife and my husband present—I barely managed to control what happened to me. I had to fight—hard—not to be treated as a routine medical emergency. They strapped me down too, and lifted my legs onto stirrups in the delivery room. Worse than that. I had to risk losing my obstetrician's good will when I refused to take an oxytocin 'challenge' test."

Anger floods me. Shame too.

"What happened?" Irene of the pleasant face, the gentle voice, is asking.

"Frédéric, my physician, got nervous when *he* decided I was late in delivering. Five days late. So I went to have the baby's heartbeat checked. It was fine. *I* wasn't fine. I had 103 degrees of fever and the New York flu. Frédéric wanted to subject me to a Pitocin test. Furious, I told him that Nature was wise enough to wait until my fever went down. Why was he so impatient? He pleaded. He insisted. I refused.

"An intern and two nurses wanted to detain me. I told Frédéric—on the phone—that I was leaving the hospital immediately. I literally ran out, as the staff looked at me disapprovingly. I took the phone off the hook at home. I collapsed. I couldn't afford to spend any energy in being angry.

"I had to be enormously sure of myself to do this. No woman should have to be so confident when she has a temperature of 103, weighs 198 pounds, and the city's covered in snow.

"Then, after thirty-one hours of hard labor, Frédéric decides I need a Caesarean. *That* I couldn't have fought. I was too weak. Too trapped. What I *did* do was push so hard when he went to get a 'second opinion' that the baby was born an hour afterward. It took me three months to recover from that final pushing. I don't think I've recovered yet.". . .

Now I'm talking. I list the matter of the Demerol "routinely" slipped into my intravenous glucose. Maybe it stopped contractions for six hours. The Pitocin slipped to me to start up contractions again. The episiotomy I never wanted. Ariel's eye infection—still!—due to the silver nitrate drops routinely given at birth. The empty or hard-to-open oxygen tank when Ariel choked at birth. The hostility toward David, the only man rooming in on the maternity floor. It's actually a long list.

I've never said this aloud before. For ten months I've kept socially silent.

"Irene," I say. "My childbirth experience was basically all right."

Why do I say this? Out of misguided respect for other women—those who had it worse? Because I don't want to appear ungrateful, unbalanced? The child lives. My feelings should be less important—right?

Do I insist childbirth was all right because it's too painful to dwell on it as otherwise? Because I don't want to admit—to myself—how powerless I am, too?

November 15, 1978

In a yellow bedroom, I'm listening to a woman friend describe her day hunting for foundation grants. I'm thinking of you, Ariel, as she talks about what we both need from the money-men. Are you still awake? Can I get home in time to see you? Suddenly Lynda says to me: "Phyllis, why don't you get a Woodrow Wilson Fellowship? You only have to be in Washington three days a week."

I reply: "Because I have a baby. And I don't want to live apart from him."

"Oh, that's right! Well then: why don't you come to our meeting on Friday about a childbirth project?"

"Because I'm working very hard, and this is too little notice. Because I can't afford to fly to most meetings, now that I have a baby."

"Oh." My friend is momentarily silenced. Into the breach I go.

"You know, Lynda, it's amazing how few women believe I have a baby. The expectation, the demand, that I be as 'free' as before persists. But no one who invites me somewhere offers to baby-sit so I can *get* somewhere or understands my reluctance to leave him home. It's impossible for me to take Ariel along with me. We're not talking about a slow walk under the sun, through dusty village streets. We're talking traffic jams, packed subway cars, riots of noise. No place to diaper him in a public restaurant. I'm not going out into *that* war with backpack and sweet maddening patience."

"Of course not," she says. Carefully. We both smile too much.

I feel guilty, incompetent, for not being able to put non-mothers, non-fathers, at their ease. Incompetent because I'm not Superwoman.

November 16, 1978

Dawn is large, lean, the mother of three children. She has ice-blue eyes that startle, that remain. Dawn photographs women in childbirth. I look at one series—and am electrified by them.

Dawn takes notes when she attends birthings. The women say: "I'm leaving." "Help me." "I want to die." "Don't interrupt me." "I can't hear you." "I can't do it."

Words we never hear. Images we're forced to imagine— or repress. Experiences not displayed in museums, not bound into books. Different experiences, different words, for each woman. I think Dawn's project is sacred.

"Who lets you photograph them?" I ask.

"Not the women who go to hospitals." She smiles, sadly. "I guess they have such shame and fear about the process that they feel a picture of it is disgusting. I've been attacked by women for wanting to do this."

Is a medical invasion of childbirth more acceptable than an "artistic "invasion"?

"I photograph women planning to give birth at home. I think that women relive their own birth passage as they're giving birth. What do you think?"

"That's a powerful idea. After all, can we ever experience someone else's birth? Even if we're giving birth to them? But why would we experience our own birth at that moment?"

Oh, Ariel: It's true, you were alone at your birth. As I was at mine—and at yours. I can only *imagine* your terror, your resolve. I was in my body, not in yours. I was somewhere on the ceiling, out of reach, out of hearing. My thoughts were in one place, my body in another.

I tell this all to Dawn.

"Yes, yes," she says. "Will you have another baby? If you do, can I photograph you?"

November 17, 1978

The sexiness of first little teeth. Yours gleam and twinkle. They make you look older.

Ariel: Where are you hiding time? I lose more and more of it each day you live.

There is no longer enough time.

To go to the movies. To get a massage. To make love. To sleep, to work. To be.

To eat breakfast.

*N*ovember 18, 1978

"I can't have any sex," Suzanne explains cheerfully. "Ever since I gave birth, it's been vaginitis, cystitis, fatigue. A month now. How about you?" It's dusk, near a stream.

"Not much sexual passion in my life," I say. "I still imagine I'm giving birth when I lie on my back. And it's ten months."

"But you're close to David. . . ."

"We're very close. Without erotic excitement. My *lover* is Ariel. His father is my brother, my mother. And maybe my son."

"Suzanne: I could use a love affair. But that's what I have with Ariel—without genital sex. Children—the secret of some women's ability to go without orgasms, or without love affairs."

"When I paint I'm often celibate for long periods," Suzanne notes, almost to herself.

"Me too, when I write."

We watch the pebbles, the smooth water.

"I feel so blessed," Suzanne confides. "To think I was ready to cheat myself of this feeling. Who ever heard of a painter-woman really pulling off motherhood?"

"Blessed is exactly how I feel." We hug. We hug again.

"We're surviving." We walk back up to the road, to the evening ahead.

November 19, 1978

"I'm getting divorced, selling the baby, running away," I inform Miriam.

"Oh, may the next seven years pass quickly," she says.

"Should I have another baby?" I ask. "Tell me how I can arrange space, the money, the right child care."

"You can't. Don't have a second. But you didn't listen to me about not having a first. It commits you for thirty-five years. No"—she laughs, correcting herself—"for sixty years. Look at *my* mother. Her children still need her. And she's eighty years old."

My mother whispers, "Have another baby—before it's too late."

"Will you help me with the twenty-four-hour child sentry duty?" I ask.

"Phyllis, I'm very tired," she says. "I'll do what I can. But you can't count on me."

"I know," I tell her.

How different is it for me, for any of us "working mothers," than for our immigrant millhand grandmothers? My work hours are as long. Like my grandmother, I can be laid off without notice. *And I only have snatches of relaxed time with you, Ariel.*

Mothers who work at home at motherhood don't have relaxed time with babies either. Who does? Does anyone?

I can't *be* with your father either. That requires elaborate planning, a baby-sitter, instructions—and then we're out on the street, tired and hungry. We have nothing to talk about but "what must be done in the house." We face each other hollow-eyed. Annoyed. Bored.

"Let's discuss the household arrangements," one of us says, finally.

"What, again?" says the other.

"Nothing's going to change. One day he'll be grown

up and gone. That's all that's going to happen."

"I can't stand it. I take no pleasure in anything. The responsibility is too much," we both say.

Then: we fight. Or we remain absolutely silent. Through dinner. Through a movie. Come home, hold each other in bed without a word, and fall asleep.

November 21, 1978

Ariel: Your father needs a haircut. His beard is bushy. He's getting thinner.

"David, how are you?" I ask.

"I'm fine," he insists. "It's nothing. It's too much," he mumbles and moves off.

He's not going to make it. His eyes gleam in despair. He's not sleeping at night. He's sleeping late in the mornings. He looks like Beth, mother of one-year-old Alexandra, across the street.

What now? A new round of interviews with "housekeeper baby-sitters" who won't clean, can't shop, and who watch television to escape from the baby? Who sit in the park, staring resolutely ahead into space, stone silent?

Where is our cheerful, bustling mother? I see her hiding in television commercials as "grandma," or as somebody else's wife.

Can she be me? *That* cheerful ever-busy person? Baking cookies, ironing sheets, gift-wrapping presents?

Baby: We've both been had. I'm not her. She wasn't born together with you, that January morning. I thought she might be: that's why I look for her. *She's missing.*

November 25, 1978

I can still see my mother at her mother's funeral: weeping, sitting alone by the coffin. I was eight. I'd never seen her cry before. How different our lives have been. She stayed home with her children and mother forever, taking care of everyone. I left her when I was seventeen.

What do I want of her? *To be with her.* I want a household arrangement of mother, daughter and grandchild. The original Holy Family. I'm being pulled into the significance of this ancient orbit.

I have more in common right now with my mother than I have with most people.

Let's speak only of our love for each other—let nothing superficial cross our lips, I'm too afraid to say. What if she shrugs it off, more afraid than I am of this resolution? She has to forgive a Persephone who *willingly* ran away, who hid from her mother, who became a "new woman."

I only have to need her again.

"Mother," I ask, "can you take Ariel overnight? Please. We need some total relief."

"No. Your brother may need me."

"He's 32 years old," I scream.

"But he's *my* baby. I have my own child to worry about," she says. "You understand," she adds. "You're a mother now."

November 29, 1978

Ariel: You're teething. You've cried all night for two nights in a row. Last night David walked the floor, Merri the night before.

This has allowed me to work today. Otherwise I'd be a shadow: dull, resigned. One sweet baby—and two people are felled by you. Things go undone that in ordinary life are easy to do, or so crucial I'd never let them slide.

Mothers tell me you're at the best age. That it gets worse as you get older. (Small babies, small troubles; big babies, big troubles.)

"I hear you," I tell them. Now I believe what mothers say. But I don't dare envision it too clearly.

*N*ovember 30, 1978

"Phyllis, how can you sit and play with him for an hour without changing his diaper? He's soaking wet. What kind of mother are you?"

David slams his books down. Loudly bangs the pot to heat your milk. I'm guilty. Guilty. I'm furious that he speaks to me this way in front of Yasmin. In front of you.

My little love: forgive me. The giggles, the laughs, so foreign to my "other" life, turned my head. No. I don't want to diaper you. I don't want to measure out the required ounces of milk, Kaopectate, paregoric. I want to play with you. Laughing deep in each other's eyes.

"Do you think he's a toy?" Your father's back. "How can I go to school and leave him alone with you? Maybe he'll starve to death."

"I did feed him," I say. "You know what? I'm not coming back! *You* support him—and yourself while you're at it."

"Pretty thick tension," Yasmin observes. "Maybe you two should have bought a hamster."

December 1, 1978

"Ba-er?" you pipe sweetly, trustingly. "Ba-er?"

"Bear!" I chime in. I surround you with them: a white bear, a brown bear, a bear cub, a well-dressed bear, a "Rocka-bye Baby" singing bear.

"Ba-er?" you still insist, without noticing any of the bears.

My fears, Ariel: If the people around you don't really respect my right, my need, to work and *not* be a full-time mother, then you'll begin to feel cheated. Not by a "society" that won't pay me—or others—for mothering. Not by a "society" that tells you myths about mothers. But cheated by me.

I fear those who teach children to respect the absent fathers, to despise the absent mothers.

Ariel: If other children all—all—have full-time mommies, you'll feel "different." One day you'll demand I stay home. You'll count my hours away.

This I fear. It will divide us—as fatefully as my giving birth to you has.

December 2, 1978

The Conference on Pornography: The male lawyer chops the air with his hand. We watch, horrified, fascinated.

"I want hard and fast evidence," he bellows. "Hard facts. Now."

Is he chopping our feminist heads off with that rigid, emphatic hand? Has he been influenced by too many pornographic movies? Hard and fast: it's everywhere.

A man. A "good" man. A lawyer who'd defend poor men, black men, Vietnam soldiers against the war. But not women. Not so fast.

I'm proud to be above you, this man's body is saying, with its deep loud voice, its fierce height, its well-dressed girth. I'm proud to be unmoved. I'm scornful of those who feel too much, who allow themselves to be influenced by soft, slow emotion. . . .

Ariel: Will you ever thunder like this? Will you lock up your woman self until she dies? Will you "operate"—surgically do a job on, kill—from your head, and never from your heart? Will you smoke pipes, unfeelingly, pompously, without humility? Will you ever harumph, surround yourself with dutiful daughter eunuchs? You, who came to me so nakedly, so trustingly?

December 3, 1978

A father stops on the street to greet your father and me.

"Man, having kids is a trip, isn't it? You learn you can adjust to anything. And survive."

His face is lined. His eyes are kind. He's my age.

"We're expecting our third in June. My oldest says if we bring another baby home she's moving out to live across the street. Good ego strength. *She's* moving. I can't concentrate as it is. I have to do my paper work at midnight, when they're asleep. But we'll manage if we have to. Even without enough space."

The philosophic perspective—if we can afford to take it—is extraordinary. The self-knowledge, strengthening.

"It goes so fast! One minute they can't talk or walk. You turn around, and they're buying the score from *Grease* and threatening to move out. It's wild!"

"Are babies sick a lot of the time?" I ask him, offhandedly. You've been sick for ten days. Again.

"Naw. My daughter is a horse. Always was. . . . Wait a minute. Every kid's different. Are you having trouble with yours?"

This father is sensitive to my unspoken question. He reassures me.

Not all men want it hard and fast.

December 4, 1978

A divorced and remarried father is speaking. Pain tightens his eyes, his jaw.

"I don't see my son very much. He only wants my money. When the child support stops, I'll probably never see him. . . . You know, my son is strange. He's a stranger too. He smokes dope, listens to music. He doesn't read."

"Did you ever want to have another child?"

"Never. Children eat your money up. They don't have that much to do with you. I can talk more easily to you than to my son. Well. He won't have my money forever."

"You mean, if he comes to you when he's twenty-five or thirty, for hospital bills or graduate school or bail, you'll say: 'Sorry, kid. My responsibility is over.' "

The father is silent.

"I don't know what I'll do. I do know this: I'm not close to him. I'm not proud of him. To get a divorce, I had to give him up. He gave me up too. You can't be a parent and live apart from your child."

We're both silent.

"I never want to experience this pain, this anger, with another human being. The disillusionment is too great. Let's change the subject. O.K.?" He manages a smile.

Can this happen to us, Ariel? I tell myself to count only on what we have right now. Your smile, your cackle, your crankiness.

I must be lying to myself. I sound magnanimous with Fate. What will I sound like when I get slapped, hard?

December 7, 1978

Last night was terrible. You shrieked in your sleep for twenty minutes. We couldn't wake you. You couldn't stop crying. Your body trembled. Your head jerked.

What if you turned blue? Convulsed? Died? You kept screaming for an hour: even after we got you up, changed your diaper. You threw the milk bottle on the floor. Rageful. Scornful. Your eyes filled with tears. You hit me, turned away.

What can it be? What would you have nightmares about? Is it gas? Is it your teeth?

Two A.M.: I'm wheeling you around in your carriage from room to room, naming objects for you. Singing to you. Suddenly—you laugh. You babble with me.

You shit.

What would I do, what would I feel, if I were alone, if your father weren't here?

Divorce is out of the question.

December 10, 1978

Child: I feel my age. No; not my age, but my poor health, my fatigue. Headaches and lower back pain plague me. My eyesight is blurred. Sometimes painful hemorrhoids. A cold constantly. I've developed a bunion. My feet ache. My breasts remain large. Too large. White hairs sprout in my head. I drink huge quantities of coffee to keep myself going. I look gray, thick-pored.

Just two years ago, when I was young, I was sprightly without enough sleep. Do you rob me of my youth? Do you rob me of the time and rest I need in order to remain healthy as I grow older?

The lab report's come back. I'm severely anemic, hypoglycemic.

I have coffee with the single mother of a teen-age son.

"Yes," she tells me. "Your body isn't ever the same again. Unless you're a ballet dancer or an athlete—or start behaving like one right after you give birth. I couldn't," she says. "Who had the time or money to be obsessive about one's own health?"

"I feel dowdy, I feel used up," I say.

"Eventually you have more freedom. That 'used up' feeling changes. But other things happen that disturb, depress."

"Like what?" I ask.

"My son is twelve now. He moves his body the way boys, men do. Where did he learn this? He's picked up less from me, physically, than from male strangers on TV. I watch him throw a ball, effortlessly, gracefully. I'm reduced to a teen-age girl watching my son. I don't throw a ball like that. So beautifully . . . "

Ariel: I pore over your photographs, taken at two weeks, and again at two months. You're very male. Your features are sensual, self-possessed. You stare quite frankly back at the camera. Proud, contemptuous. You remind me of Bronzino's Young Prince.

December 12, 1978

Women say to me, in 1978: How can you do this to him, how can you deny yourself this pleasure, how can you let him grow up with strangers, you'll be sorry later, it passes so fast, he won't know you, can't you slow down, work less hard, I had to slow down, I don't regret it, it's worth it, it's terrible, it's wonderful. . . . *Don't dare be different or I'll hate you. And punish you if I can.*

Hazings. They're hazing me. Without pity. Without looking into my trapped and wounded eyes. Without seeing themselves there.

Why don't they keep quiet? Why are their voices so loud? Why do I listen to them?

One of the voices is your grandmother's. Hers alone pierces my resolve.

Ariel: We must do things a little differently, a little sanely. I cannot drown in you.

December 15, 1978

Ariel: I want to run away. I want only the desert stars, silent and huge, for companions. I want an attic room in Amsterdam. A bicycle, a café.

I need a permanent vacation from crushing responsibility. Even at my age, it's too much. *Especially* at my age.

It's the whole grind, grinding me exceedingly fine.

I dream of mythical full-time motherhood. I imagine starring with you in a commercial. There I am, stirring the pudding, testing the roast. The kitchen is yellow. It is always afternoon. We are always happy. You are about five years old. Forever. We seem to be alone, like the mother and child in the TV advertisements for pie crust or detergent. A neighbor, a plumber, stop in, but never to stay. Your father—absent, like the Heavenly Father.

I'd need a sewing room for migraine headaches.

I'd need a curving staircase for throwing myself down.

I'd need my own locked bathroom to hide the liquor, the pills, the cookies in.

O fat-bottomed one! Where should we run to?

December 22, 1978

With your coming, I am both provider and lover, child and mother. I'm ferocious on behalf of your survival. Therefore I'm gentle, and very emotional.

I am without the traditional signs and symptoms of a "maternal instinct." I don't shop for your bananas or mash them myself. I don't take you to the pediatrician. I don't agonize when someone else—your father, or Merri—are with you, "in my place." I'm not sure I have a set place: as your personal nurse-maid or full-time companion. *If I do, I don't want it.*

(Am I being tricked out of "having" you by the patriarchal demands of my career? Am I being cheated of you by my need to earn money or to write books? Is there some organic twosome we should be growing into—lest you die, lest I be revealed as monstrous, unfit?)

Baby: Maybe. But I think not. I notice this: You don't cling, terrified, to any one of us (yet). You take comfort from each of us.

You stop everything to listen to me sing operatic arias to you. Your eyes grow round with pleasure. Laughing, you fathom my animal imitations. Crawling fast, you want me to overtake you, clattering loudly, while you shudder in pleasure. Over and over again.

When Merri comes in, her coat still on, you pound your bottle, you shriek in anticipation of the games you'll soon be playing. You scream, "Here I am, ready! I haven't forgotten what we two do together."

You smile and smile when your father's near you. He soothes you out of crankiness into sleep. Clearly, here you're king: sitting atop his shoulders, swung way up in the air.

You grab, hold onto the hair on our three heads with equal mania, sucking your thumb, eyes closed in happiness.

You accept the round of part-time baby-sitters. Without

long introductions. You play with each one. You let yourself be fed. You fall asleep easily.

And sometimes you want me—me, specifically—not to leave you. And I don't. I stay. How I stay.

December 23, 1978

Naming this book is harder than naming you, Ariel. I choose and discard a title every hour. *Unnatural Mother. Inside Out. Mother-Longings. Spinning Miracles.* You *are* a miracle. I've spun you into being. The dictionary describes our last twenty months together expertly.

> **spin.** to make (yarn) by drawing out, twisting, and winding fibers. . . . to produce a thread from the body, as spiders, silkworms, etc. . . . **spin off,** to create something new. . . . to produce, fabricate, or evolve in a manner suggestive of spinning thread: to spin a tale of sailing ships and bygone days. . . .
>
> **spin.** to cause to turn around rapidly. . . . as on an axis; twirl; whirl. To move, go, run, ride, or travel rapidly; . . . to have a sensation of whirling; reel: My head began to spin and I fainted. to revolve or rotate rapidly. . . . as the earth, a top, etc.
>
> **spin.** a downward movement or trend, esp. one that is sudden, alarming, etc., Also called **tailspin, tail spin.** *Aeron.* a maneuver in which an airplane descends in a vertical direction along a helical path of large pitch and small radius at an angle *dangerous when not done intentionally or under control* (my italics).

Ariel, I looked up *spiral* thinking of our double helix, and found an aerodynamic description of maternal ambivalence.

> **spiral** *n.* 1. *Geom.* a plane curve generated by a point moving round a fixed point while constantly receding from or approaching it. . . . *adj.* 8. running continously around a fixed point or center while constantly receding from or approaching it; . . . 9. coiling around a fixed line axis in a constantly changing series of planes . . .

I am without a title. What's in a name anyway?

December 24, 1978

"Can you help with Ariel for a week?" I ask my mother.

"I can't live with you," she says quickly. "I'm not comfortable in somebody else's house. I like to know where everything is. He can stay here, with me."

"I won't be able to visit him if he's two hours driving time away. Let's compromise."

"Then keep him altogether." She laughs. "It's your responsibility. Not mine. Let it be your pleasure too."

"Mother, David has five exams next month. I have a writing deadline. We haven't been able to find a full-time baby-sitter for the month. We've even run out of time to look for one."

"So you really need me! But not for a week. I can't promise I'll be up to it. What if I don't feel well? What if your brothers need me? I can only try."

It will be like this always. My mother will never be my willing servant, my approving parent. But we will always begin again. One of us will call the other, act as if nothing has happened.

December 29, 1978

"Mother, how long were you in labor with me?" I ask, drying the dishes.

"Why do you ask?" She bristles, moving the plates more swiftly now.

"I want to know. I was there too." I plead.

"No you weren't. I was totally alone."

Confirmation from my mother.

"I think it started at one or two in the morning," she says. "You were born in the early afternoon. I had to wait for your father to take me to the hospital. He worked nights then. But it's not important. Why dwell on something that hurts?"

"It's very important," I tell her. Then why have I never asked her before? And why am I comparing our number of hours in labor? Me: thirty-two and a half. My mother: twelve at most.

"It was very traumatic for me," she continues. "I cried for days. I cried for my mother. It made no sense. But this is very private. Why do you want to know such private things?" she asks me for the one hundred thousandth time since we've met.

"Do you know I searched for you all through my pregnancy . . . and still do?"

"You left me long ago," she jeers. "I don't trust you. But here I am. Still."

She looks me over: Torn pants. Scuffed boots. Limp hair.

"You know, you look like you need a mother." She laughs.

And now she does something extraordinary. She takes an eyebrow pencil (where has she hidden it?) and starts to draw a better eyebrow line on me. She, who doesn't wear make-up. Doesn't approve of it. She—my maker—is still improving, touching up her handiwork.

"I don't know if we could live together," we both say.

Both dreaming of it.

December 31, 1978

"No one knows you're my daughter," she says. "You're always busy. I don't understand what you're busy doing. You don't take care of your husband, your house, your child."

"Where did you go wrong, Mother?" I ask. Lovingly.

She's saying what she's always said. But I'm hearing it differently. *I'm hearing how much she wants me to be exactly like her.*

"I want you to be a housewife," she bursts out. She's finally said it. "Why not? Promise me you'll think about it. . . . Also, we're never alone. Why can't I see you alone? Why can't you stop working and stay home with your precious, precious baby?"

Triumph is mine! She loves me! She loves me! Only she wants me to be exactly like her. Otherwise she won't believe I love her too. I fled this deadly merging, this oneness, long ago. To avoid it, I have gone motherless for thirty-four years.

"Let's make a date. Alone," I propose. "How about next weekend? Saturday night?"

"Don't you have to be with your husband? Don't you think you should check with him first?"

Oh, my precious mother. No. No, I don't. My freedom is so dazzling it blinds you. The price I pay for it would set you to weeping.

I'll tell you about it. Someday. Maybe.

January 1, 1979

When I became your mother, Ariel, people sent cards, then stopped calling. Friends, colleagues, still invited me out: as long as I behaved like "myself": as I was before I gave birth.

For a year now, I haven't seen ten close friends. For a year I've asked myself: Am I imagining this? Is it my fault? *It can't be related to my motherhood.*

Ah, but it can. Suddenly I've been demoted to another category. One from which I cannot rise: except from my own ashes.

I say "demoted," not "promoted," because I feel the most overwhelming and subtle loss in social status since I've become a mother. I might never have know this if I wasn't "something else" first.

After eighteen years of my being an adult among other adults, only your father is really involved in our fragile new-born family.

Most people I know are merely indifferent. The new mothers, the new fathers descend like me, each alone, screaming.

Ten million new parents, each alone. It's crazy. It's unbearable, says my friend Alta.

It is.

Epilogue

January 6, 1979

Last year I died. My life without you ended. Our life together—only nine months!—ended too: abruptly and forever, when you gave birth to me. Being born into motherhood is the sharpest pain I've ever known. I'm a newborn mother: your age exactly, one year old today.

I've dropped ten thousand years down an ancient well. My own life threatens to peel off: insignificant, recent. My stomach knots, my nails redden, to break my fall. Screaming.

I write this book to chart my descent. To slow my descent.

And to thank you for coming. Little ancestor, sweet baby! How you temper me, deepen me, like an ancient smithy working slowly. You—who need everything done for you—are the most powerful teacher I've ever known.

Last night, lying in a hot, white-foamed tub, I was suddenly pregnant with you again. I wept, aware that you no longer sleep beneath my heart.

It was you—Ariel!—in there, in me. I didn't know that. Will I grow sad every year in winter, when you leave me to be born?

This soft belly, rounded still, with your footprint. Proof

of your origin, your passage through. Here, here is where you walked, without setting foot to earth. Your first moon, little astronaut.

Because of you, I'll return to Earth, transformed: no longer a virgin, but a mother, married to a child.

Together we have engaged in alchemy.

Know, Ariel: We have always been separate. While I was pregnant. During labor. From the moment you were born. Always I had some sense of your utter separate reality.

And who could be closer than we two?

Other Books to Read

A bibliographic survey of all the writing during the last ten thousand years about the experience and consequence of pregnancy, childbirth, and motherhood doesn't exist. I lacked the time—the precious time—to create one.

This list of books is not a scholar's list. It is one woman's list of books that were relatively easy for me to buy, order, or borrow—books that comforted and inspired me.

Alta. *Momma: A Start on All the Untold Stories.* New York: Times Change Press, 1974.

Arms, Suzanne. *Immaculate Deception. A New Look at Women and Childbirth in America.* Boston: Houghton Mifflin, 1975.

Barber, Virginia, and Skaggs, Merrill Maguire. *The Mother Person.* Indianapolis: Bobbs-Merrill, 1975.

Bernard, Jessie. *Self Portrait of a Family: Letters by Jessie, Dorothy, Lee, Claude and David Bernard.* Boston: Beacon Press, 1978.

Bernikow, Louise, ed. *The World Split Open: Four Centuries of Women Poets in England and America, 1552–1950.* New York: Random House, 1974.

Bing, Elisabeth, R.P.T. *Six Practical Lessons for an Easier Childbirth.* New York: Bantam Books, 1973.

Boston Women's Health Book Collective, The. *Ourselves and Our Children: A Book by and for Parents.* New York: Random House, 1978.

Broner, E. M. *Her Mothers.* New York: Holt, Rinehart Winston, 1975
———. *A Weave of Women.* New York: Holt, Rinehart & Winston, 1978.

Broner, E. M., and Davidson, Cathy N., eds. *Mothers and Daughters in Literature.* New York: Frederick Ungar, 1979.

Chodorow, Nancy. *The Reproduction of Mothering: Psychoanalysis and the Sociology of Gender.* Berkeley: University of California Press, 1978.

Curley, Jayme, et al. *The Balancing Act: A Career and a Baby.* Chicago: Swallow Press, 1976.

Davies, Margaret Llewellyn, ed. *Maternity. Letters from Working Women.* London: G. Bell and Sons, 1915; Virago Limited, 1978.

Demeter, Anna. *Legal Kidnapping: What Happens to a Family When the Father Kidnaps Two Children.* Boston: Beacon Press, 1977.

Dinnerstein, Dorothy. *The Mermaid and the Minotaur.* New York: Harper & Row, 1972.

Ehrenreich, Barbara, and English, Deirdre. *For Her Own Good: 150 Years of the Expert's Advice to Women.* Garden City, N.Y.: Doubleday & Co., Anchor Press, 1978.

Fallaci, Oriana. *Letter to a Child Never Born.* New York: Simon & Schuster, 1976.

Gilman, Charlotte Perkins. *Women and Economics.* New York: Harper & Row, 1966.

————. *The Living of Charlotte Perkins Gilman: An Autobiography.* New York: Harper & Row, Colophon Books, 1975.

Goulianos, Joan. *By Woman Writ: Literature from Six Centuries By and About Women.* Indianapolis: Bobbs-Merrill, 1973.

Griffin, Susan. *Woman and Nature: The Roaring Inside Her.* New York: Harper & Row, 1978.

Hindmarch, Gladys. *A Birth Account.* Vancouver: New Star Books, 1976

Jong, Erica. *Half-Lives.* New York: Holt, Rinehart & Winston, 1973.

————. *Loveroot.* New York: Holt, Rinehart & Winston, 1976.

————. *At the Edge of the Body.* New York: Holt, Rinehart & Winston, 1979.

Jordan, Brigitte. *Birth in Four Cultures: A Cross-Cultural Investigation of Childbirth in Yucatan, Holland, Sweden, and the United States.* St. Albans, Vt.: Eden Press Women's Publications, 1978.

Kingston, Maxine Hong. *The Woman Warrior.* New York: Alfred A. Knopf, 1976.

Lazarre, Jane. *The Mother Knot.* New York: Dell Publishing Co., 1976.

Maroger, Dominique, ed. *Catherine The Great. Memoirs.* London: Hamish Hamilton, 1955.

Marzollo, Jean, comp. *9 Months 1 Day 1 Year: A Guide to Pregnancy, Birth and Babycare.* New York: Harper & Row, 1976.

McBride, Angela Barron. *The Growth and Development of Mothers.* New York: Harper & Row, Perennial Library, 1973.

———. *A Married Feminist.* New York: Harper & Row, 1976.

Morgan, Robin. *Monster.* New York: Random House, 1972.

———. *Lady of the Beasts.* New York: Random House, 1976.

———. *Going Too Far.* New York: Random House, 1977.

Olsen, Tillie. *Tell Me A Riddle.* New York: Dell Publishing Co., 1961.

———. *Yonnondio: From the Thirties.* New York: Delacorte Press, 1974.

———. *Silences.* New York: Delacorte Press, Seymour Lawrence, 1978.

Ostriker, Alicia. *The Mother/Child Papers.* Feminist Studies, 1978.

Paley, Grace. *The Little Disturber of Men.* New York: Bantam Books, 1959.

Pildes, Judith. *Our Mother's Daughters.* Berkeley, Calif.: Shameless Hussey Press, 1979.

Plath, Sylvia. "Three Women: A Poem For Three Voices." In *Winter Trees.* New York: Harper & Row, 1972.

Quest: A Feminist Quarterly, vol. IV, no. 3 (Summer 1978).

Radl, Shirley L. *Mother's Day Is Over.* New York: Warner Books, 1973.

Rich, Adrienne. *Snapshots of a Daughter-in-Law.* New York: W. W. Norton, 1967.

———. *Of Woman Born: Motherhood As Experience and Institution.* New York: W. W. Norton, 1976.

———. *Diving into the Wreck.* New York: W. W. Norton, 1976.

Roiphe, Anne Richardson. *Up the Sandbox.* New York: Fawcett, 1970.

Rush, Anne Kent. *Moon, Moon.* New York: Random House, 1976.

Sexton, Anne. *All My Pretty Ones.* Boston: Houghton Mifflin, 1962.

Shulman, Alix Kates. *Memoirs of an Ex-Prom Queen.* New York: Bantam Books, 1973.

Smedley, Agnes. *Daughter of Earth.* Old Westbury, N.Y.: Feminist Press, 1973.

Spock, Benjamin. *Baby and Child Care.* New York: Pocket Books, 1976.

Thornton, Alice. "The Autobiography of Mrs. Alice Thornton," in *By a Woman Writ: Literature from Six Centuries By and About*

Women. Edited by Joan Goulianos. Indianapolis: Bobbs-Merrill, 1973.

Viva. *The Baby.* New York: Alfred A. Knopf, 1975.

Walker, Alice. *In Love and Trouble.* New York: Harcourt, Brace, 1968.

Wittig, Monique. *Les Guerilleres.* New York: Avon, 1972.